LEARN MORE ABOUT THE BENEFITS OF MEDITATION

Meditation is an art that has been around since the dawn of the age of man. This is not a statement to be brushed over. After all, many many things about mankind have changed over time, but the profound art of meditation is something we have clung on to dearly. This is because there is no substitute for meditation. Nothing else, single handedly, bestows the many wonderful blessings that meditation brings... in fact nothing else even comes close. In this article I will outline the top 10 benefits that meditation brings and hopefully it will inspire all to learn and practice this timeless art.

The mind of one who meditates is like the easy, leisurely flow of the Ganges River, as compared to the ordinary mind, which is like Niagara Falls. In other words your mind is at peace, deeply silent and so you are at peace.
Meditation opens up the channels of communication between all levels of your being. What this means is that you have access now to the guidance that is coming directly from your Divine Self.

This link gives rise to the flow of intuition and wisdom.
Meditation strips away the layers of false identity that mask your True Self from shinning through. Once you eliminate these false egos and stop catering to their nonsense you can reside in your True Nature. This brings forth joy and happiness as it allows you to be at ease with life, existence and yourself.
All serious meditators know how much their brain function has been enhanced by meditation.

Now, empirical studies every day are indicating this link. Meditation will undoubtedly increase your awareness and will significantly increase your intelligence.
The parts that are not put on but are natural. This will give you insight into who you really are and what you really love in life. That is the secret of mastering the art of living and discovering your true talents, gifts and purpose. That which you love, you do for its own sake without the need for reward of accolades. Once this is discovered, life can be lived with passion, zeal and independence.

Enlightenment: This is the one ultimate purpose of meditation. To help you discover the True Non-Dual Nature of Reality. To make you realize that your True Self is Divine and One with God.

All serious meditators know how much their brain function has been enhanced by meditation. Now, empirical studies every day are indicating this link. Meditation will undoubtedly increase your awareness and will significantly increase your intelligence.

Take your time and practice meditation today so that you can start feeling better real soon. This is going to be a life changing experience for you if you can make the most out of it and really start being a much more positive person, there is no doubt about that. Now, empirical studies every day are indicating this link. Meditation will undoubtedly increase your awareness and will significantly increase your intelligence.

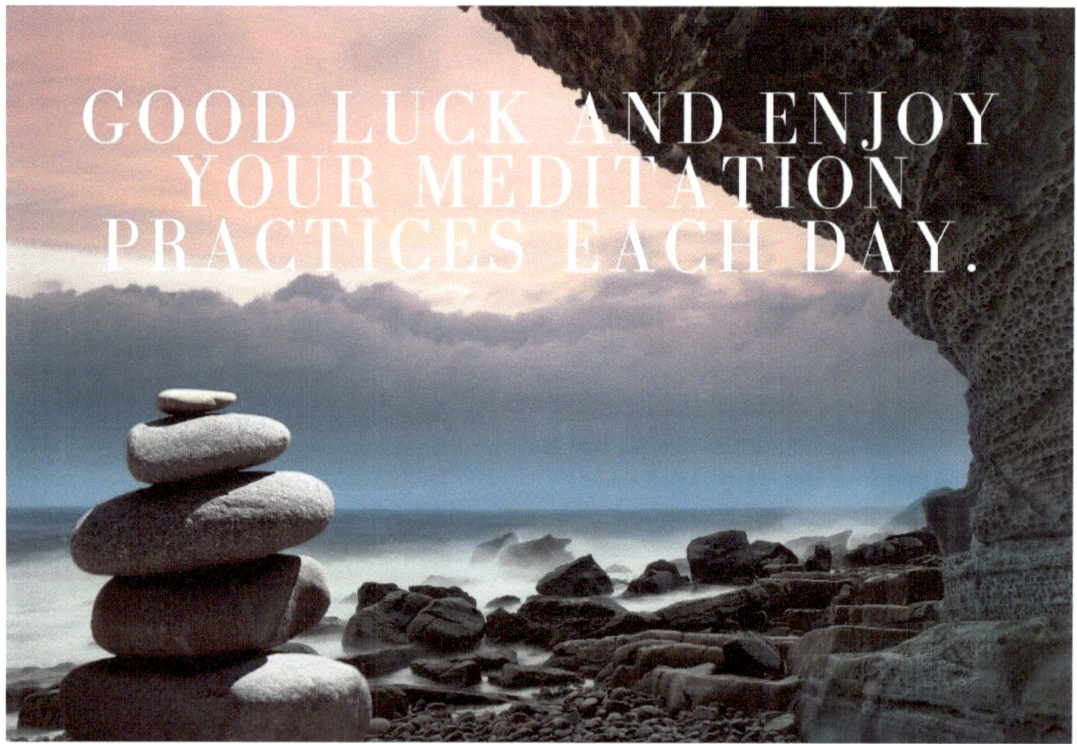

GOOD LUCK AND ENJOY YOUR MEDITATION PRACTICES EACH DAY.

THINGS TO KNOW
ABOUT MEDITATION
THAT MIGHT HELP YOU

Meditation is easy to do and can give you an instant feeling of calmness and relaxation.

This mediation technique is simple and very effective and only takek you a few minutes to learn and will help you relax away from the stresses of everyday life.

A definition accepted in most dictionaries for meditation is, continuous and profound contemplation or musing on a subject or series of subjects of a deep or abstruse nature. Meditation can provide you with inner strength and you are going to be much happier.

This is really reflection.

Meditation generally involves where one consciously discounts wandering thoughts and fantasies, and calming and focusing the mind, while controlling the breath, and sensory awareness.

There is one meditation anyone can do, and by doing it, one's life force itself comes under control; ones senses turn off, and the mind becomes quiet. Then the peace and realization that comes from true meditation comes to the practitioner.

What is the name of this meditation, and how is it done? Even spoken over and over, the syllables merge...so one is saying Sohamsoham...I am He, He am I...it is a prayer and a meditation mantra which are spiritually charged word or series of words used a meditation theme.

One feels close ones intuition, and one feels as if the world of material things is less important due to its overbearing insignificance when compared to the bliss one feels in meditation.

Sit up straight with your spine in a line...do not slouch.

ou must be comfortable, so sit on a chair or on the floor with a soft mat or carpet underneath you.

When you feel completely relaxed, command your mind to be silent, your emotions to be still, keeping your body as relaxed as possible.

As you do this meditation, actually imagine the air entering your nose and traveling all the way down into your lungs. This is one So.

As you exhale, you can imagine the air traveling out of the lungs, up to the nose and out of your body. This is one Ham.

Beginners in this meditation usually silently say the word So with each inhalation and the word Ham with each exhalation. Continue in this way, as long as you are comfortable, but no less than 5 minutes, and no longer than 20 minutes until the meditation feels natural to go longer.

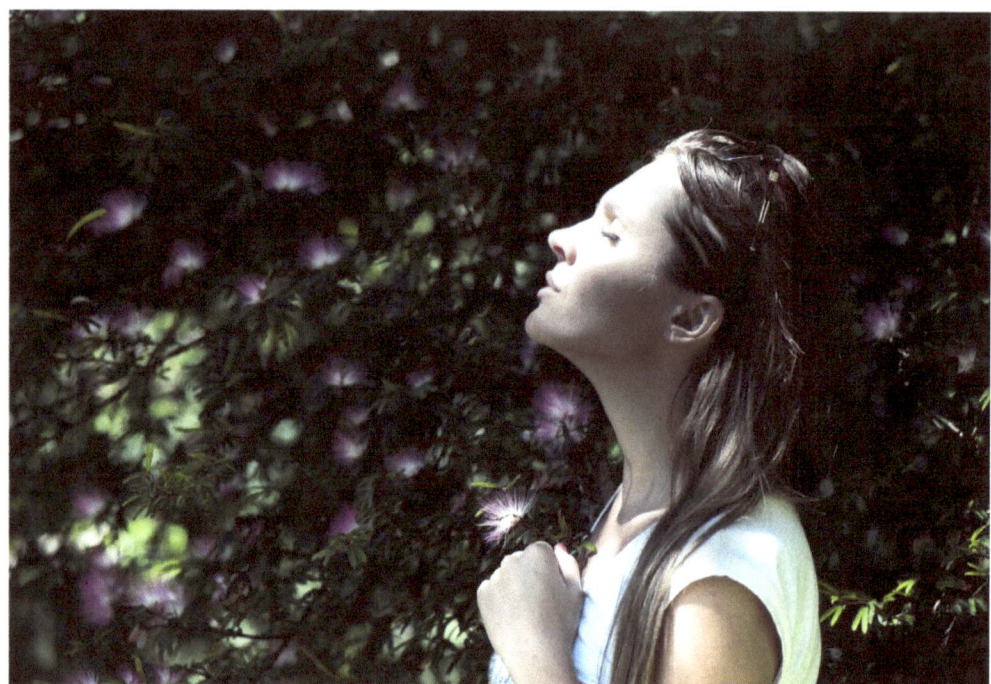

A definition accepted in most dictionaries for meditation is, continuous and profound contemplation or musing on a subject or series of subjects of a deep or abstruse nature. This is really reflection.

Meditation generally involves where one consciously discounts wandering thoughts and fantasies, and calming and focusing the mind, while controlling the breath, and sensory awareness.

This mediation technique is simple and very effective and onlu a few minutes to learn and will help you relax away from the stresses of everyday life. Learn as much as you can about meditation so you too can start feeling better.

MEDITATION CAN HELP

As you exhale, listen to the sound and associate it with the word Ham. As a guide, So sounds as does if you are saying it in English. Ham could actually be written as Hom, as the in Ham is very weak.

Meditation is one of the most important spiritual disciplines. The benefits of regular meditation are numerous, too many to list, yet peace of mind is one of the greatest.

Try listening to our Let Go recording (see holisticmakeove m link below) which utilizes brain-mind technology to effortlessly guide you into a meditative state.

Avoid all drugs. Even "just" marijuana "only once in a while" hinders intuition and clouds your mind for weeks afterwards.

Try meditating with someone you love or with a group of friends. The combined energy will help you go deeper.

You may be sensitive to something you're eating or drinking. Pick a day and eat lightly, perhaps about half of what you usually do. Consume what you know will be easy to digest, such as lightly steamed vegetables.

You should be able to focus more easily provided you feel lighter and more alert. Certain supplements, herbs, and medications, especially if they affect your mood, may be disagreeing with your system and causing you to be scattered. Ask your doctor or health professional for alternative recommendations or if you can do without them for a while. If you keep asking God or your guides or angels of the Light how you can be more successful with meditation, you'll eventually become aware of effective ways to go deeper and focus better.

You'll be a pro in no time.

If you're still having trouble perceiving anything, jump start the process by using your imagination. Tell yourself you'll perceive the first image, thought, or feeling, in response to any of the questions or instructions in the script, on the count of three. Then count one, two, three and provide a picture or thought from your imagination or memory. Continue this process until other images that feel more related to the issue you are exploring start filtering into your mind.

Try relaxing music. Experiment with different kinds to test which works best for you.

Whatever works the best for you is what you should be thinking of trying out. Meditation can change your life for the better and once you begin feeling better you will know that you definitely made the best choices by choosing this to help you along the way throughout this difficult life.

Learn more about meditation the next chance that you can because your life will be ever changing because of it. There is more to be learned about it even to this day. Things are going to be different in your life and meditation can be the reason for your healing and becoming a much more positive person that is happier and healthier.

The internet is the best place to locate information about meditation, and there are many wonderful websites that could provide you with tons of information.

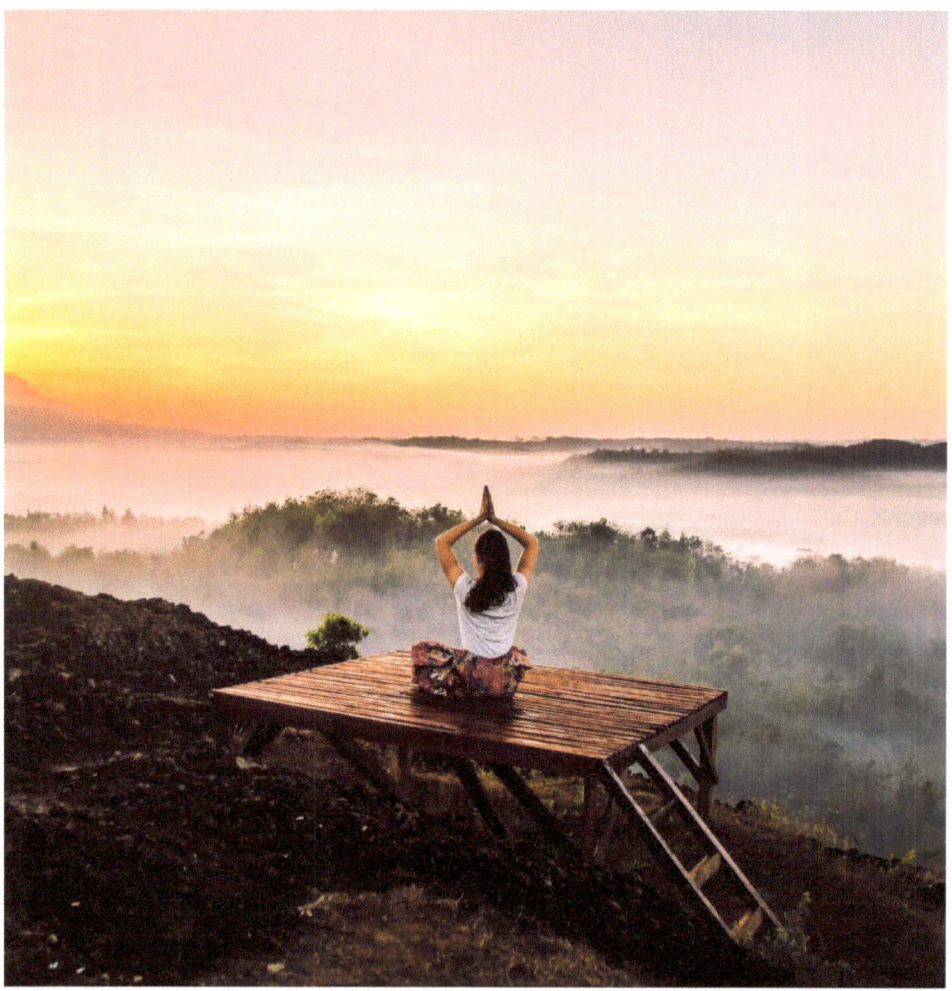

TECHNIQUES THAT YOU MIGHT NOT KNOW ABOUT MEDITATION

Meditation and holistic living have become buzzwords in recent years, with more and more people seeking an alternative to the frantic pace of modern life. However, many practitioners don't consider the barriers modern society presents to meditation. Even seasoned meditation practitioners can lose focus in the speed-crazed, mindset of modern life. Meditation encourages a strong self awareness and a healthy mind-body connection. Today's culture seems to operate on a completely different system.

The modern world is addicted to activity, and the more the better. Because of this, many people remain chained to distractions and cannot tap into their body's natural potential to break free.
Stress is created when the mind is not doing what the body is. If you are doing bills and your mind is wandering from picking up the kids and making dinner to finishing up at work, that creates stress. But if your mind is focused on what your body is doing, then there is no stress. This is a fundamental meditation technique.

Most meditation techniques assume the mind-body already exists. This works well in a mountain monastery, but can be difficult to achieve with the hectic pace of modern lifestyle. A more basic gateway into that mind-body connection is needed. A transition from the modern world into meditation should tap into the senses. You're trying to strengthen the bond and focus your attention on multiple levels. Look for ways to utilize textures that interest you, sounds that soothe you, and scents that enhance your focus.

Experiment with simple, easy motions to relax your body and to prepare yourself for meditation. Motion can focus the mind and help you break away from the whirlwind of thoughts generated each day. Think of running your hands through a river, or through a fountain if you have one available. Play with smooth stones, or make shapes of clay or sand. Flip a smooth stick of wood or roll it back and forth between your hands.

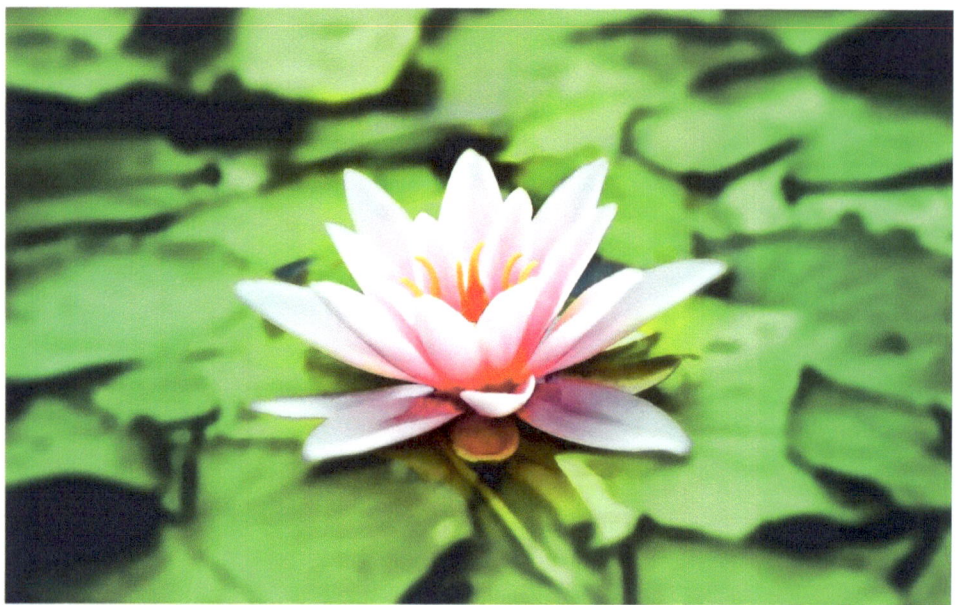

Once you've disconnected from the modern world, you can truly take advantage of your meditation time. A more centered, aware state of being will allow you to delve deeper into your inner self. You might be surprised at what you can see with eyes unclouded.

Once thought of as a ritual performed by men who shaved their heads, wore long robes and lived in a mountain cave, this mind quieting, stress relieving natural self-healing practice is becoming so commonplace that corporations such as Deutsche Bank, Google and Hughes Aircraft recognize the intuitive powers of it and offer meditation classes to their employees.

Having the ability to quiet one's mind and retreat to a thought-free state of calmness opens the connection to higher intelligence and greatly enhances problem-solving abilities. In addition, with practice and coaching you can develop the ability to ask pointed questions and receive answers to them through this same dynamic channel.

The number of miracles born out of a regular practice of meditation are untold. From loosing weight and quitting smoking, to manifesting more money and physical items, to rekindling relationships and curing terminal diseases, millions of accounts of miracles just like these are attributed to meditation.

MEDITATION IS SOMETHING ALL OF YOU SHOULD KNOW MORE ABOUT

Guided meditations are one of the best ways to start meditating.
They're simple to use, which if you're in need of relaxation is a helpful reason in itself.

Probably the hardest thing about using a relaxation meditation is actually making the time to listen to it.
That may sound odd, but we tend to place least priority on ourselves. We look after others, help others and generally do our best to help them to lead better lives.

Set aside the necessary time. If you think you can't find the time, think again. There are almost certainly times in your day when you can find 20 minutes or so. Cut out watching the news for starters - that will have the beneficial effect of keeping you away from negative influences as well. Find a comfortable chair if you're going to listen to your guided relaxation whilst sitting down. Or find a bed to lie down on if that's the position you'd prefer.

Finding the time is far and away the most difficult part. And even that's easy when you set your mind to it.
Put on your headphones. If necessary, put a "do not disturb" sign on the door to your room.

Press play and let your mind wallow in the stress-free luxury of listening to a guided relaxation.
Finding the time is far and away the most difficult part. And even that's easy when you set your mind to it.

Then switch the cell phone to silent.It's actually really simple to use a guided relaxation meditation to relax yourself.

Meditation is something that any one of you out there could practice at any stressful time in your lives and it will really help matters not seem so severe. There are many different books on the internet where you could learn more about meditation and start practicing it each day. This is important for you to do in order for you to feel better about your situation in life.

Read through many different magazines and books until you truly understand what meditation can do for you in your life, it is really going to improve every single aspect of it, there is no doubt about that. There are ways of feeling better through meditation but if you do not push yourself to do so then you are going to be one very unhappy person at the end of the day.

Meditation can save your life in many ways because of the changes that it will make you feel each and everyday that you step out of bed. Tell your friends about it and they too can benefit from practicing meditation everyday that they wake up or before going to bed. This is something positive that you can do for yourself and for your mental well being for many years to come.

Do some sort of meditation everyday for a couple weeks and just see how much better you feel about things. It is going to really surprise you alot.

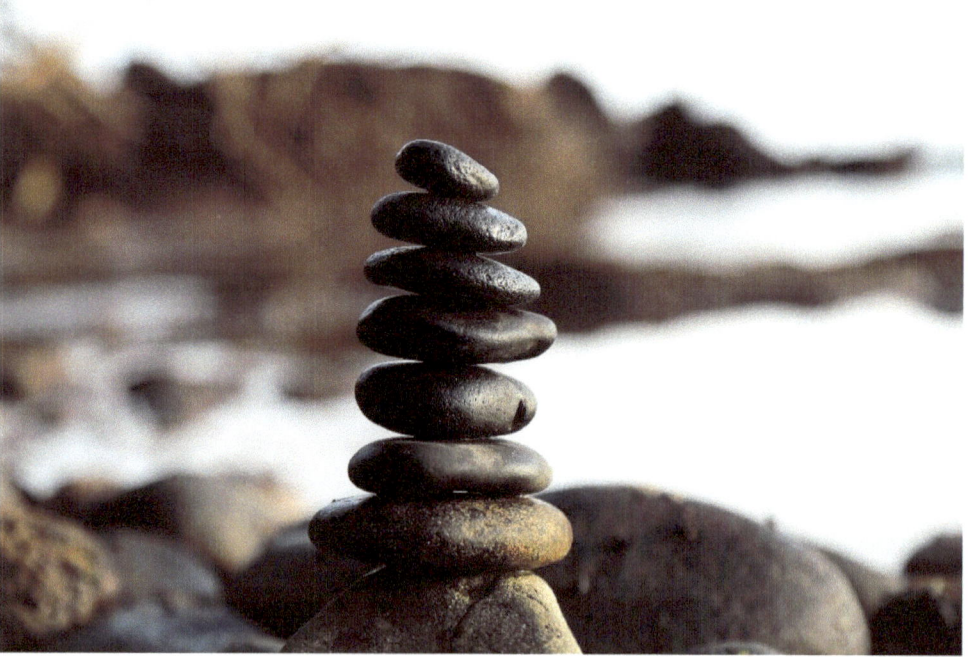

METHODS OF MEDITATION TO IMPROVE YOUR HEALTH

We all know there are many different methods of meditation to help relieve stress and to relieve tension and relax you. The first thing you want to do is remember that there are ways to meditate that will fit your lifestyle. You may have a friend that has used meditation to help them relax and would want to give you advice on how they meditate. You must realize that the person you are talking to has a whole different lifestyle then you do.

Your friend can suggest ways that help him or her but will it help you? If you are an active person exercise can be a very good and healthy way to meditate. Walking can be very relaxing and it can give you time to gather your thoughts while getting healthy at the same time. If you are not the kind of person that is not use to a lot of exercise and you feel walking would help you meditate make sure you start out slowly. Do not try and walk 2 or 3 miles starting out. You want to meditate but you want to relax while doing it. If you are not use to exercise you do not want to ware yourself out.Walk slowly and take time to gather your thoughts.

One of the most relaxing ways I find to meditate is by prayer. I will be the first to admit I do not know a lot about the bible and probably do not actually pray in the way that most people do who know a lot about the bible. My point is I want to relax and have time to myself by meditating and I take my comfort in the lord. I guess you can say I talk to the lord more than I pray. Meditation can really turn your life around.

I actually feel that me talking from my heart is the same as saying a prayer from your heart. I remember my mother would take the prayer list from church and no matter how many peoples names were on the list she took the time to sit and meditate and say a prayer of healing and comfort for each and everyone on the prayer list. My husband finds he can meditate and relax by listening to music.

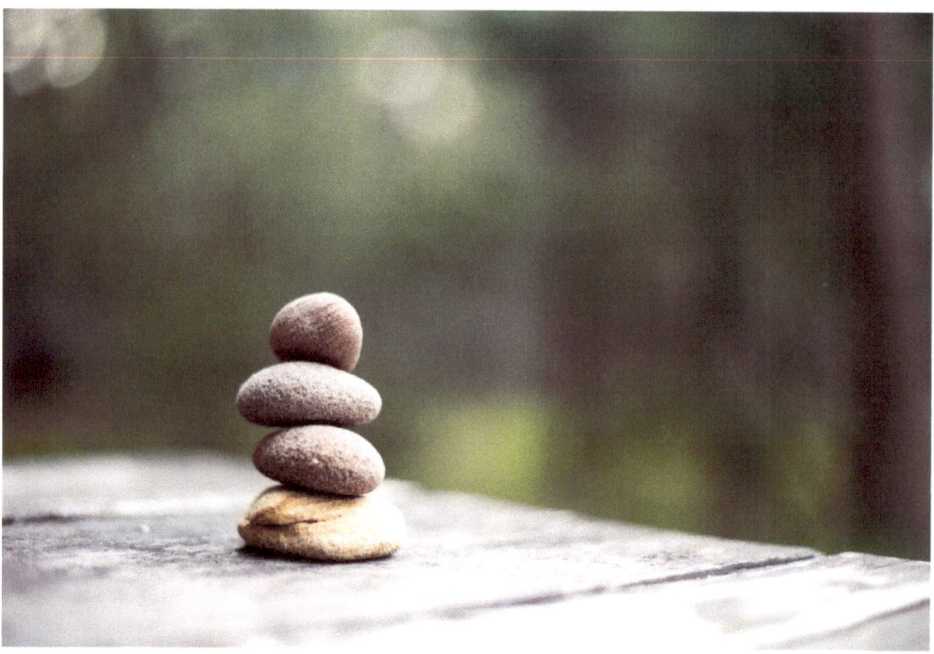

He actually has hundreds even thousands of different types of music he listens to. His nerves are not really good so his comfort is in his music and he plays the radio day in and day out. He mostly listens to classic country and the oldies station. The music helps him concentrate and keep his thoughts together.Another way I find of meditating is through animals.You can talk to your pet without worrying about him talking back to you like a child would.

You can curl up on the couch turn the television on low and just communicate with your pet. You may think how do you communicate with an animal? Animals are very smart. They understand what you are trying to do. If you have had a bad day they can comfort you by just being there for you.If you have a dog or a cat let them sit or lay next to you and pet them and you will be so relaxed you will forget about the stress your day has brought.

So whether you are meditating by a method of exercise, or a method of communicating with your animals or by prayer take the time to just relax your mind and your body and you will be physically and emotionally stress free. Remember meditation is basically taking the time to collect your thoughts and when you take the time to get your thoughts together your mind will then be able to concentrate on the things that are important in your life.

METHODS OF MEDITATION TO RELAX YOU

We all know there are many different methods of meditation to help relieve stress and to relieve tension and relax you. The first thing you want to do is remember that there are ways to meditate that will fit your lifestyle. You may have a friend that has used meditation to help them relax and would want to give you advice on how they meditate. You must realize that the person you are talking to has a whole different lifestyle then you do.

Your friend can suggest ways that help him or her but will it help you? If you are an active person exercise can be a very good and healthy way to meditate. Walking can be very relaxing and it can give you time to gather your thoughts while getting healthy at the same time. If you are not the kind of person that is not use to a lot of exercise and you feel walking would help you meditate make sure you start out slowly. Do not try and walk 2 or 3 miles starting out. You want to meditate but you want to relax while doing it. If you are not use to exercise you do not want to ware yourself out.Walk slowly and take time to gather your thoughts.

One of the most relaxing ways I find to meditate is by prayer. I will be the first to admit I do not know a lot about the bible and probally do not actually pray in the way that most people do who know a lot about the bible. My point is I want to relax and have time to myself by meditating and I take my comfort in the lord. I guess you can say I talk to the lord more then I pray. I actually feel that me talking from my heart is the same as saying a prayer from your heart.

I remember my mother would take the prayer list from church and no matter how many peoples names were on the list she took the time to sit and meditate and say a prayer of healing and comfort for each and everyone on the prayer list. My husband finds he can meditate and relax by listening to music. He actually has hundreds even thousands of different types of music he listens to. His nerves are not really good so his comfort is in his music and he plays the radio day in and day out. He mostly listens to classic country and the oldies station.

The music helps him concentrate and keep his thoughts together.Another way I find of meditating is through animals.You can talk to your pet without worrying about him talking back to you like a child would. You can curl up on the couch turn the television on low and just communicate with your pet. You may think how do you communicate with an animal? Animals are very smart. They understand what you are trying to do.

If you have had a bad day they can comfort you by just being there for you.If you have a dog or a cat let them sit or lay next to you and pet them and you will be so relaxed you will forget about the stress your day has brought. So whether you are meditating by a method of exercise, or a method of communicating with your animals or by prayer take the time to just relax your mind and your body and you will be physically and emotionally stress free.

Remember meditation is basically taking the time to collect your thoughts and when you take the time to get your thoughts together your mind will then be able to concentrate on the things that are important in your life.

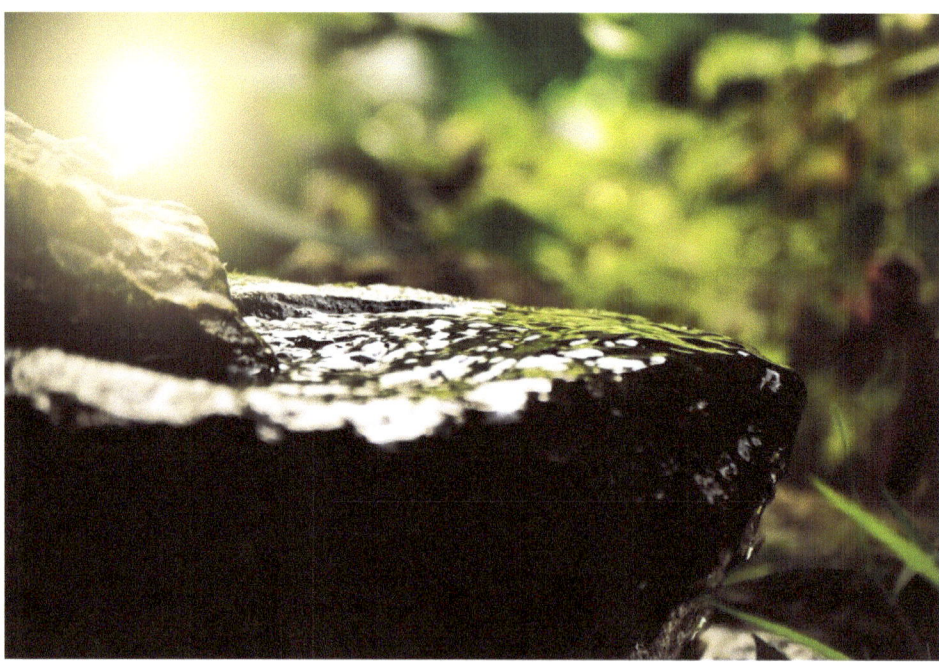

HOW TO RELIEVE STRESS BY MEDITATION

The word meditation simply is defined as to be in a continuous contemplative thought or to simply just think about doing something. We all have different types of stress in our lives. Some of us our stressed out over a job,or maybe a relationship,or children,or if you are like most of us you are stressed over finances. Taking the time to meditate in your own relaxing way will help with the stress you are feeling.I have learned that worrying about what is stressing you will not help solve the situation that is upsetting you.

You may think that taking time out of your already busy life to meditate is ridiculous,But it is not ridiculous it will absolutely help calm your nerves which will help you relax enough to sit down and calmly work out the situation that is upsetting you.I found that I can relax and meditate by sitting and relaxing in a hot bubble bath.If you are worried about not having enough time to sit and relax in a hot tub maybe you can just go outside for a breath of fresh air and take time to just collect your thoughts. After everything has calmed down you can then take the time to take a hot relaxing bath.

If the kids are stressing you out you know how easy it can be to lose your temper with the kids,So things don't get out of control you can do breathing exercises to help meditate you. Let the kids go outside for a few minutes or maybe let them watch a movie or whatever they like to do within reason for a few minutes so that you can get your thoughts together when meditating.Breathe in and out slowly and take time to think about what options you have to control the situation that has upset you. With having to deal with our children,our jobs,our relationships,and our finances it's a wonder we all can even go on every day.

Find a way of meditation that will work for you and you will see that even if it's for only a few minutes that will be a few minutes you don't have to worry about things.If you don't want to go on the Internet to find ways to relax then go to your library in your town. There will be many,many books on relaxation by meditation. When you are in a place like the library you can actually just relax in that environment where it is quiet and relaxing. Get you 2 or 3 books and find the one that will help you the most.

You know you can also write down notes on the other books you have read. Maybe check out a couple of books that talk about different ways of meditating and write down the chapters that interest you the most. Even if you start out by just learning how to have peace of mind that is a very big accomplishment. After you have found peace of mind you can then start working on the daily things in your life that has left you feeling empty inside. Remember you can have the life you have dreamed of if you just take the time to learn ways to help you with relaxation techniques. You can find fulfillment in your life and defiantly make a difference in your life and the lives of others who feel the pressures of every day life.

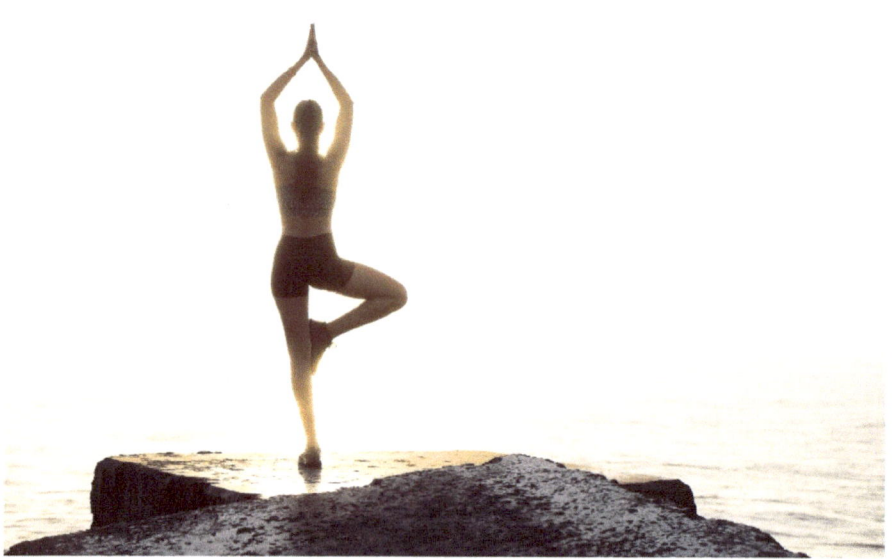

Whether you find meditation and relaxation techniques through books,tapes,or even exercises you will find that when your life is free of every day stress you can then start to find solutions to the many different problems in your life in a calm peaceful way. You can go on line and find self help tapes about meditation. Do you want to just settle on a life that can make you miserable day after day? You may feel so empty inside that you feel as if you have no purpose in life.

You have to remember you are using your thoughts in your mind to meditate so you want to take the time to clear out all the negative feelings you have in your mind so that you can concentrate on how to improve your life and make a goal for yourself. Meditation can help. When you take the time to relax and really stop and think about things that are going on in your life you can also find that you are relaxed enough by meditating to find solutions to many different things you question in your life.

HOW MEDITATION CAN HELP YOU STOP SMOKING

Is it true that meditation can help you quit smoking? Have you ever thought about it? Can we possibly do something that easy to make you stop smoking? Everything is possible. What I am going to tell you in this article is what I have found. What you can do to stop smoking.

Meditation has long been considered as one of the very few ways by which man could access himself without really having to accommodate the intervention of the logical mind. Meditation helps relieve the stress of everyday life and it helps the person rejuvenate his mind to function more effectively. Apart from these, meditation is also considered as a cure to some diseases and disorders, especially those that are infiltrated mostly by stresses.

When people meditate you become more relaxed and clam about your everyday life. Some people smoke more when they are stressed. This is a proven fact. People often chain smoke because they are under stress. Your mind becomes weak from stress resulting to the deterioration of the body and the will to continue what was first a goal. So there for when someone is constantly stressing and if you just take a second or however long you want, begin the process of meditation.

We already know that the cost of smoking is very expensive. When you smoke more than one pack a day, the cost that you are spending is very high. You probably do not realize that within a years time you can probably spend almost half of your earnings on smoking. Just think what you could have done with that money if you found what could help you stop smoking. Meditation could be one of the methods that could help you stop smoking.

Meditation to help quit the smoking habit acts in many different ways. The person from the pressure of temptations but on the other hand, the person will be rescued from the pressure of not being able to meet the goal. The former conceives the smoking cessation on a much brighter side since meditation could help drive the person with complete motivation to stay quit even when the mind calls for a last smoke.

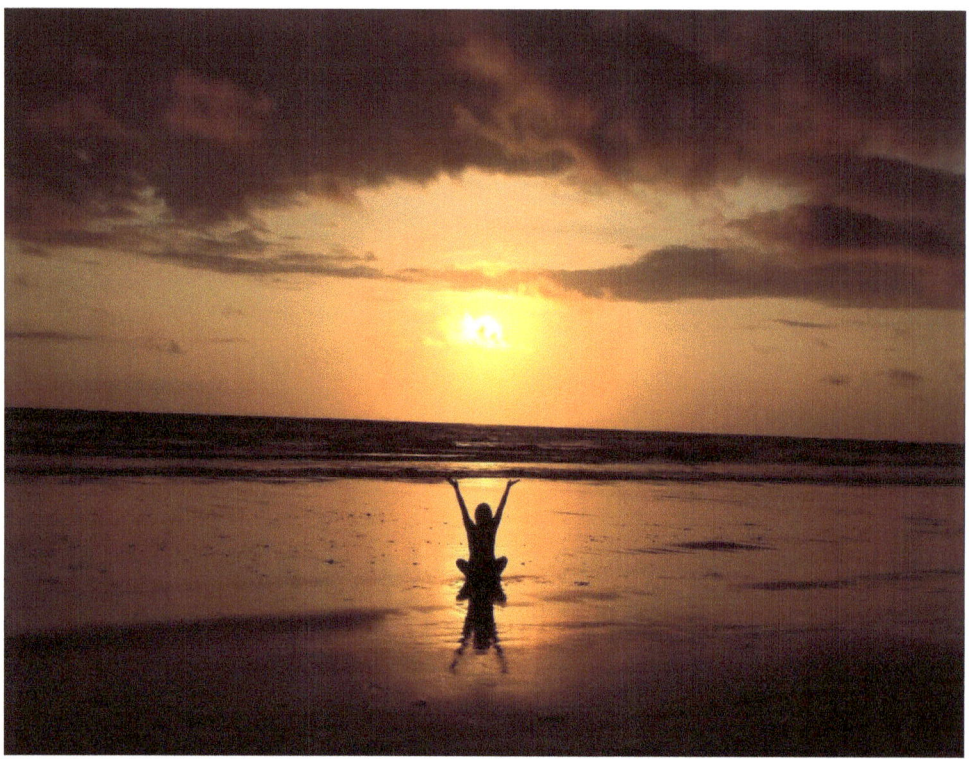

They say quitting smoking is one of the hardest habits to quit. You have to put your mind into it. If you do not have your mind set to something then it will not be a focus. Meditation can help you get that mind frame that you are looking for. You have to take many things in consideration when wanting to quit a bad habit. It is very stressful and sometimes you will not succeed on your first try, but do not give up. There are other ways out there.

If you find out that meditation is not the way for you, then there are many other options out there you can find. Contact your local doctor or research it online. There are over the counter medicines out there you can try. You just have to find out what works best for you.

HOW KARATE CAN HELP WITH MEDITATION

Although the ancient origins of karate are somewhat unclear to us, The one thing I can tell you, is that about 1400 years ago, while teaching at the Shaolin Temple in China, Daruma Daishi used techniques that were similar to karate. Later these techniques developed into forms of karate known as Shaolin Boxing.

You need a clear mind to use Karate and meditating is the best way to clear your mind when you are in a sport such as karate. In 1955 one of master funakoshi's last direct pupils cam to the United States and was the first person to teach karate in this country. That same year he put together Southern California Karate Association, which has grown over several years to now become a national non-profit organization.

As I meditated I continued to learn more about karate. I learned in 1961, which happens to be my year of birth, Mr Caylor Adkins, One of Mr Ohshima's first black belts, began attending CSULB and soon formed the school's first karate club. In 1968 after being gone for a while he returned to CSULB along with a gentleman named Mr Don Depree. Mr Depree carried on the tradition and led the growing club until the year 1992, when he entrusted the leadership of the club to Mr Samir Abboud.

Still keeping my mind clear by meditating I learned that Mr Samir Abboud was a continuing student of Don Depree since the year of 1969. Samir was the CSUBL captain of the karate club, and assistant instructor to Mr Don Depree for many years. Through meditation children and adults learn breathing techniques that help them concentrate on karate. When first starting karate you will want to start with the beginners belt. The purpose of this level is orientation.

Students will be taught the general structure of the class, basic commands, the importance of self-defense and some basic combinations of self-defense moves. By concentration with meditation the student will learn to be familiar with and to perform any of the moves on the curriculum sheet. The students also should be able to stand in a Chunbi position for 1 minute without moving. Minimal proficiency will be required.

The practicing time 5-10 minutes 3-4 times a week will be plenty for the beginners level. It will usually take 4-6 weeks to start your next belt. So whether you are a child or and adult learning karate for whatever reason, remember the key to karate is first using your breathing techniques and your meditation will help you to practice your breathing.

Meditation books are also very helpful, if you are interested in learning more about meditation just go to your local library and check some of them out. Take time out to study meditation and you could be feeling much better real soon, which is something that most of us all want for ourselves. Good luck and remember that keeping a positive attitude can really make a difference in your stress levels. Please take time out for yourself for meditation.

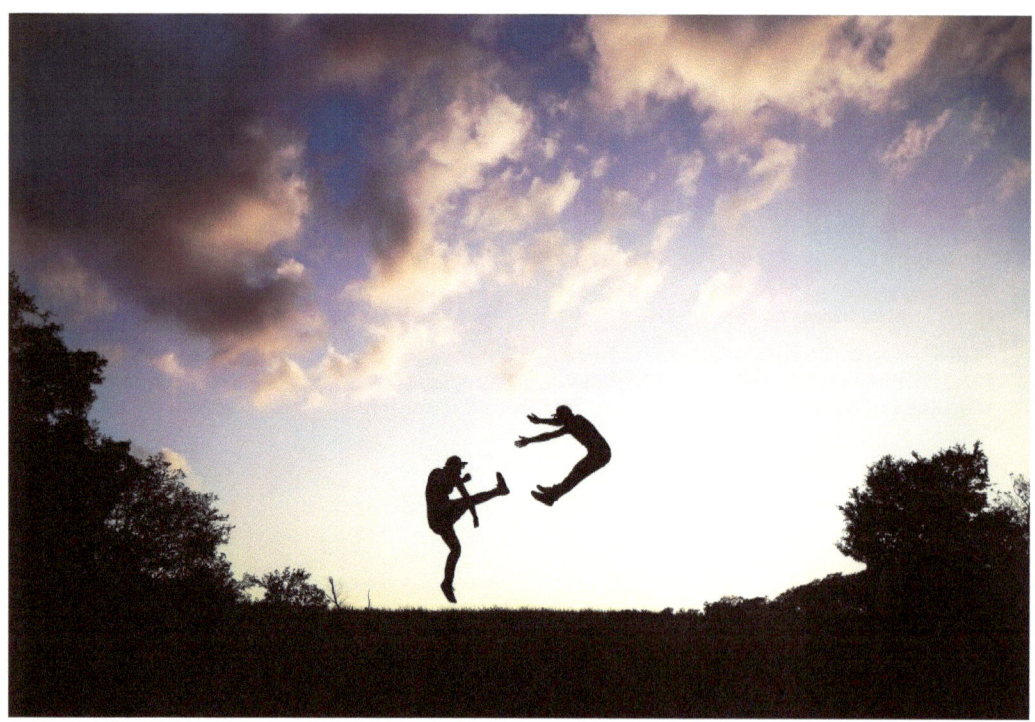

HOW MEDITATION HELPS INSOMNIA

Insomnia simply is a chronic inability to sleep. I have had many restless nice with only a few hours a sleep. Many nights I would only get 3 or 4 hours of sleep. I had tried everything to help me sleep.I tried things like Tylenol pm.mild nerve pills and even was tested for sleep apnea and had a breathing machine to use at night for the sleep apnea.That machine made me feel as if i could not get any oxygen. Insomnia can make you crazy after awhile.

I was having a very difficult time breathing with it. I had to quit using the machine because it was so uncomfortable.I was getting very irritable from not sleeping so a friend told me how using mediation helped her.I went on the computer and found out many ways meditation helps people for many different problems. The first thing I learned is that having insomnia can also be a mind thing.

You can actually train your mind to go without sleep.I know that I think about the struggles I go through everyday and keep that on my mind so I cannot sleep well. Through meditation I have learned to calm down,relax and know that getting so upset over things I cannot change will just make things worse. Now when I come home after a exhausting day I don't let things bother me so much. I actually first started my mediation in the morning before I left and again when I get home.

In the morning I get up about 30 minutes earlier then the rest of the family so I can have time to myself. I go into the kitchen get a book I like or a newspaper,fix me some coffee and just meditate before I have to start my hectic day. When I come home at night I know that with my insomnia I will have another restless night so I start preparing for my night after I get supper cooked the dishes done and kids to bed.

For my meditation at night I will first relax by listening to soothing music. I will turn on a music channel on my television and just kick back and relax. I then get in a hot tub and sit there and let the hot water sooth me. After I get out of the tub I do not wait to go to bed. Since my body is now very relaxed I go straight to bed. I have learned by staying awake watching TV after I am so relaxed will only make it harder for me to sleep.

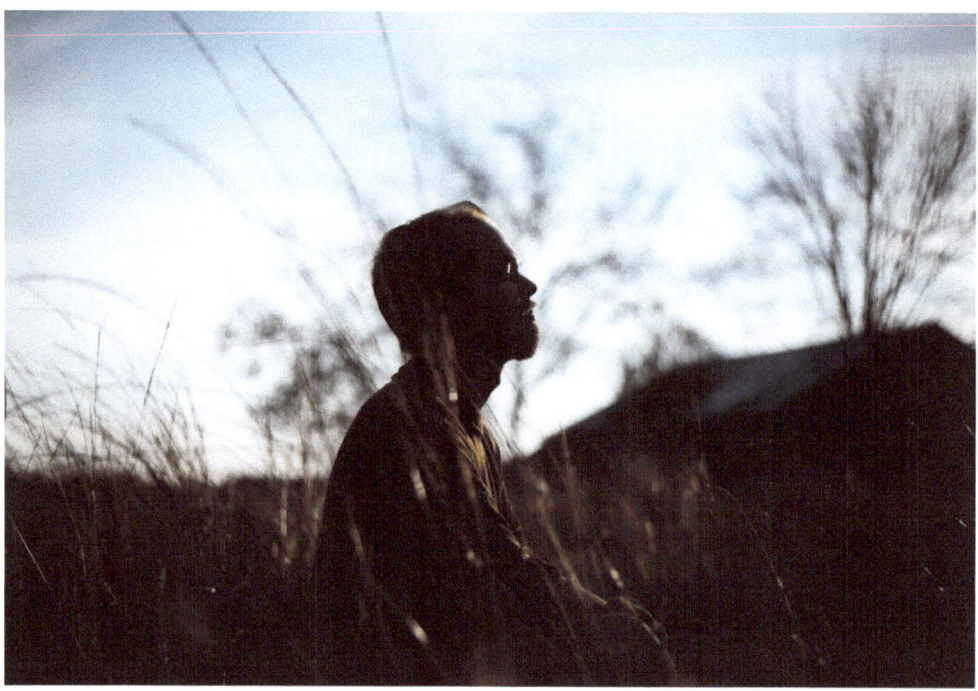

Since I used my meditation while listening to comforting music and relieving my tension with a hot bath why get upset by watching television. I turn my fan on low get under the covers take some deep relaxing breaths and go to sleep. I'm not saying that I am cured and get 8 hours of sleep every night but I can say that using mediation to relax me has helped me at least get a couple of extra hours of sleep then I use to.

My husband also turns on the little clock radio to a country channel and leaves it on low all night to help him get some sleep. You have got to remember meditation is simply clearing your mind of thoughts that upset you. Once you have cleared your mind over whatever is bothering you it will be to your benefit.

Relaxing is the key to having a better day and night. So find a way of meditation that will help you relax and just enjoy your night. You are worth it and most of all after all you do for everyone you deserve to have a few moments of relaxing meditation.

MEDITATION- EXPLANATIONS ABOUT IT

For sufferers of insomnia inability to relax physically and mentally well enough to sleep is often a problem. Thoughts race and make it difficult to shut down and get to sleep until it is nearly time to get up again. The nightly routine of fighting with a racing mind in hopes of a few minutes of unbroken sleep becomes their routine. This article was written to give insomniacs tips as well as advice that is geared toward falling asleep easily. Meditation will always be beneficial.

The first thing we need to do in this battle against insomnia is discuss the problem with your doctor. Often there is a medical reason behind sleep difficulties. Staying away from sleeping pills is the next thing you should do. Sleeping pills can cause addiction problems as well as add other issues that can cause insomnia defeating their purpose. Sleeping pills also impair mental acuity. Placebo studies have shown patients who were given a placebo actually slept better and were more refreshed than those who were given sleeping pills.

After that you need to keep in mind that there in not a quick-fix for insomnia. While there may be instances that popping a pill can take care of the problem; insomnia isn't one of those instances. There can be many reasons for insomnia which sleeping pills wouldn't address, and chemically induced sleep is not as refreshing as the real thing. Having a routine will also help you to get enough rest as well as keep insomnia at bay. If you keep track of when you go to bed and when you get up for several days you will most likely find a pattern. Often insomnia can be treated by setting a schedule and following it while watching your sleep patterns. You need to be exposed to natural light daily as well.

Going outside to get natural sunlight is also important. You need sunlight for over-all health in addition to stabilizing your sleep patterns. Meditation can improve sleep, you can also try listening to soft music in the evening to help you relax. Daily exercise is important for the brain as well as the body. Exercise can help you relax and ensures a deeper, more restful sleep. It is a good idea to have a dark, cool, quiet place to sleep with a comfortable and well supported sleeping surface. You should sleep in your bed instead of in a chair reclined in front of a television set.

Start your sleep period by relaxing your body starting with your toes and working your way up until your whole body is relaxed. Proper diet plays a large part in sleep habits. You need to get enough vitamins and minerals, especially calcium and magnesium. St John's Wort can improve mood if you are suffering from depression, which commonly occurs in people with insomnia. Ginseng and Ginkgo Biloba can help with concentration during the day as well. Before starting any supplements you should seek the advice of a licensed medical professional and through meditation.

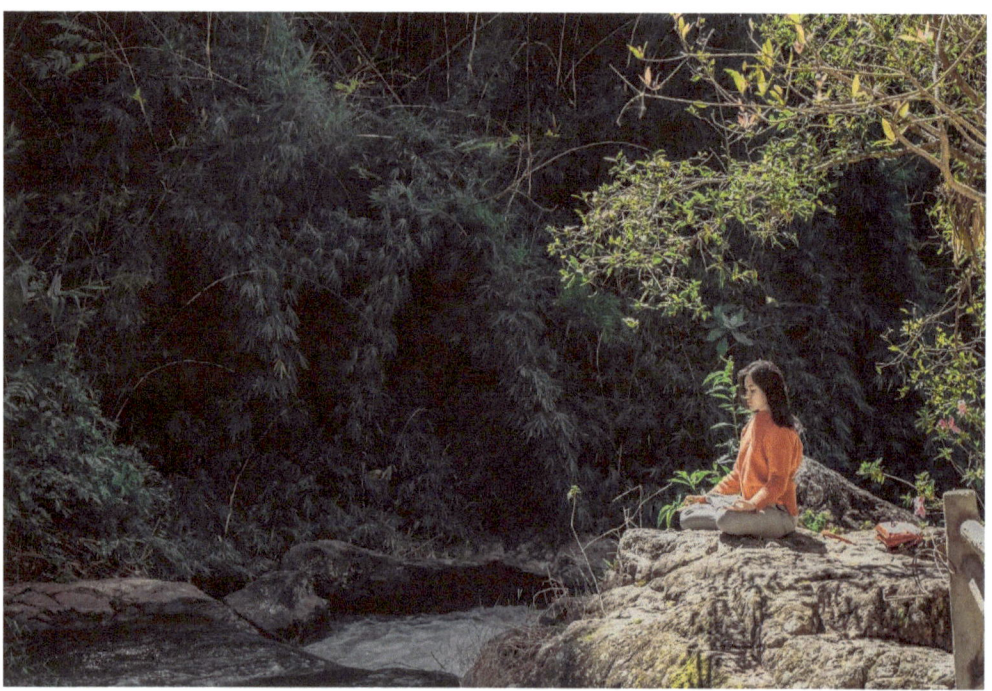

MEDITATION THROUGH PRAYER

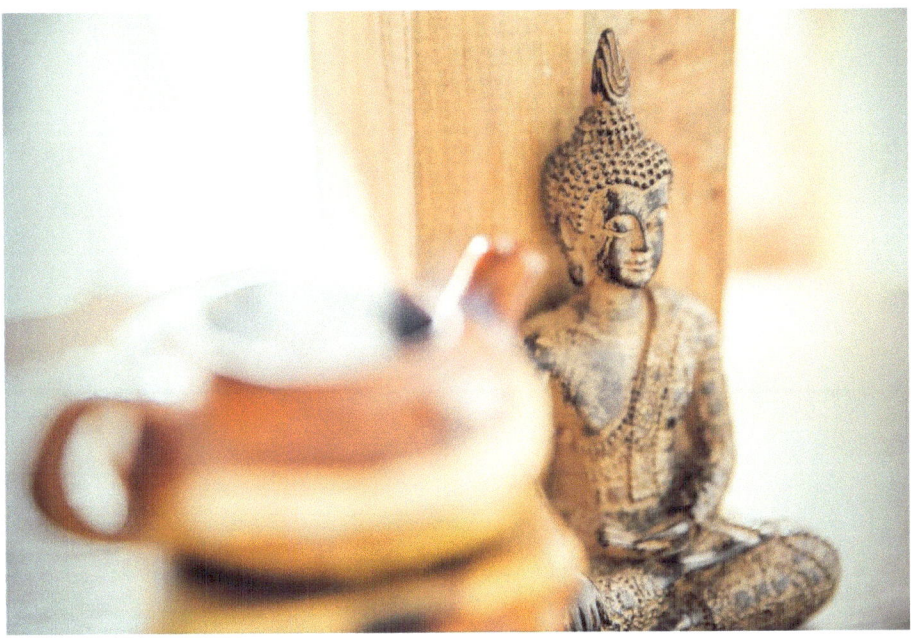

I know there are a lot of us that pray for people who are sick,or maybe someone that has lost a loved one,or for peace in the world,or maybe you even pray for a lost soul.Whatever it is you may pray for you do it out of the love and faith you have in your heart.Meditating through prayer just gives me a peaceful feeling inside.I guess you can see that when I pray I don't pray like maybe a minister would pray.I know all about god,however I will be the first to admit I do not know a lot about the bible.

I understand the meaning of what the bible says but I do not understand a lot of the words.I basically should say I use meditation to just talk to god.I believe that the way I talk to god is the same way that people may pray to god. I went to church today and the minister was talking about another minister that liked to tell everyone he knew about everything he has done good in his life. He bragged so much that he really didn't have the time to listen to what the people in his church needed. I guess you could say even though he preached an excellent sermon and did everything a minister should do,He just really couldn't see that his pride was taking over his life.

After meditating for a few seconds are minister went on to tell a story of a very religious Christian man and a tax collector walked into a temple at the same time.You could tell when the tax collector walked in everyone stayed away from him because he was not well liked.The Christian man prayed that he would not ever turn out to be anything like the tax collector.The tax collector said a simple prayer asking god that he may be worthy of gods love.I'm sure the Christian man did a lot of good things in his life,But maybe he should have meditated about his pride.

The tax collector did not look down on anyone or asked god if he could be like someone else,he just asked to be worthy of gods love.We all have done things that we wish we could take back.We pray that god will forgive what we have done and we then feel better about ourselves.We know god can forgive us but the important thing is can we forgive ourselves.We truly cannot be happy with ourselves until we do.

I am very concerned about someone I love very much right now.She is a very good Christian person,also a very hard worker and is very sick. She never complains and has been through very much and will have to continue to go through a lot.

As I was meditating in church I felt the tears coming and all I could do is ask god over and over again to please lay his healing hands on this person I love very much. So whether you are practicing meditation through prayer to heal someone you love or to have peace in the world I can tell you the prayer you are saying will comfort you and give you peace of mind.

MEDITATION USING YOUR BODY AND BRAIN

There is a constant two-way communication going on between your body and your brain.Do you remember a time when you may have thought of something that was just terrible or maybe you had a "sinking feeling" in your stomach area? That is the kind of communication that goes on between your brain and your body.Meditation can help relax your mind so it can help train your body to relax and your brain to be clear.

Recent research has found that not only does your brain communicate with your cells,but your cells will also communicate with your brain and also with other parts of your body.In fact,scientist have recently discovered that we think with not only are brain but our bodies as well.Meditation can help us to also understand about our brain.It is not inaccurate to look at your entire body as being part of your brain.

That may be a new fact that may startle you,but do not reject it.Many scientists are now starting to believe that we are actually a "bodybrain".You can communicate with your body and brain through meditation.A key part of your body's incredible communication system involves your cells' receptors.This means every call in your body can have millions of receptors on it's face,and each cell has perhaps seventy different types of receptors.

While meditating as I learned more I discovered that in the early 1970s,Candace Pert,PhD.D, was the first scientist to prove that the existence of these receptors with her own discovery of the opiate receptor.This receptor molecules float on the cell's oily outer part of the membrane and also have roots that can reach deep inside the cell.I'm sure that Dr.Pert had to do a lot of meditating as she wrote her wonderful book The Molecules Of Emotion,Dr.Pert says that "the life of a cell,what it is up to at any moment,is determined by which receptors are on its surface,and whether those receptors are occupied by ligands or not.

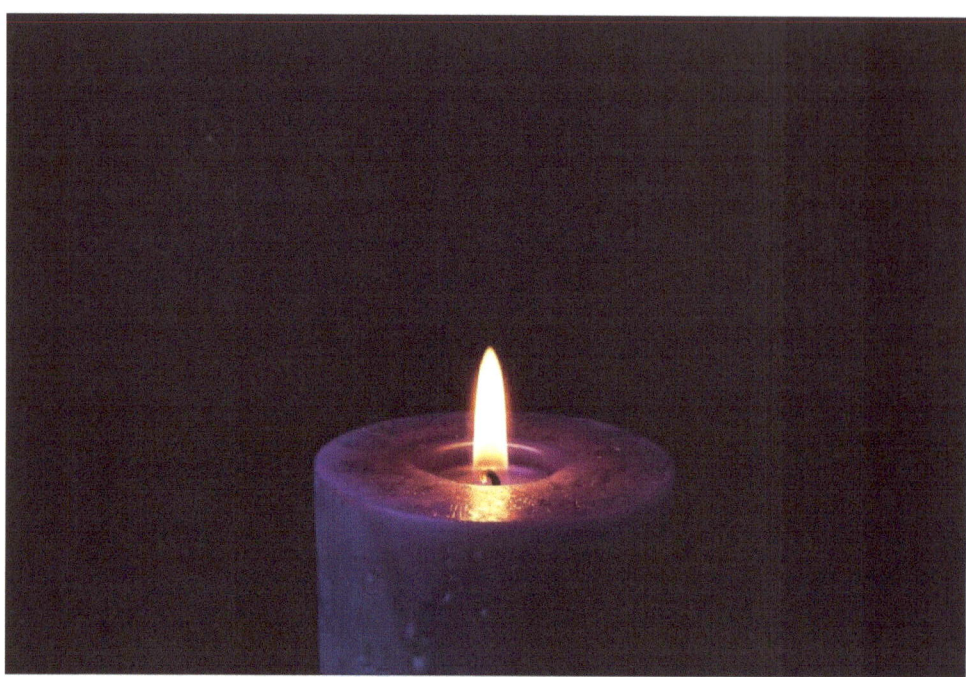

A ligand is described as a small molecule that will bind itself to a cellular receptor. Still using mediation to keep my mind clear I learned that there are three chemical types of ligands. They are the neurotransmitters, the steroids, and the ones that we are most interested in at this time, the peptides. According to Dr. Pert, as many as 95 percent of all ligands may be peptides.

The receptors and their ligands have come to be seen as "information molecules'- the basic units of a language that are used by cells throughout the organism to communicate across systems such as the endocrine, neurological, gastrointestinal, and even the immune system." I would say as much knowledge as Dr. Pert has on this subject meditation would be what kept her mind in focus.

HEALING YOUR PAST WITH MEDITATION

We all know it is not possible to roll back time or undo or change bad decisions we made in the past,however using meditation we can change the way we feel about the bad decisions we made in the past so that they will stop tormenting us here in the present. We all carry a lot of baggage from the past,such things as maybe a broken heart,hurt feelings,or bad memories of friends or loved ones that have lied,cheated,or betrayed us,events that may have brought us pain,or we may torment ourselves over opportunities we may have missed out on or even wrong choices we made in our lives.

We absolutely cannot allow ourselves to let things in the past we cannot change take over our present lives.Meditation is simply collecting our thoughts in a relaxing atmosphere.If you take the time to learn how to heal your past it will enable you to be happy in the present. You may ask how can you heal the past? You can look at past situations you cannot change in a brighter light with a new understanding on the events in the past have hurt you.When your by yourself in a quiet place start your meditation.

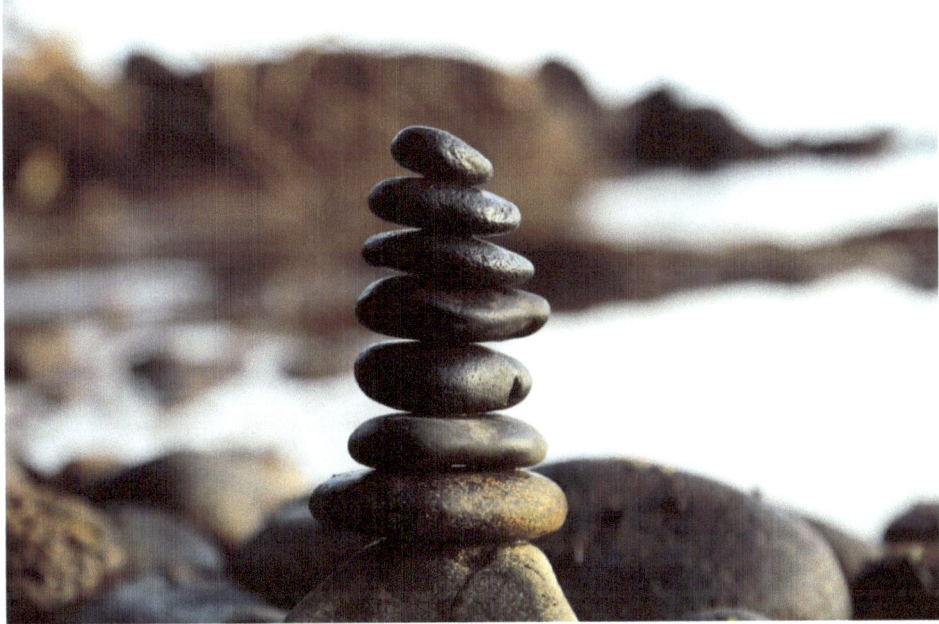

Think about how whatever may have happened to you in the past may even be a benefit to you.You know how bad you felt when something or somebody said or did something to you that you felt that you had no purpose in life or was not good enough to associate with others.Meditating about how those things in the past made you feel helps you to understand how others who are now in the same situation you were in then feel about themselves.

You know how they feel so you maybe can tell them your experience back then and how you turned it around and made a life for yourself.So many of us just need someone to take the time to just say hello or nice day isn't it? Just a kind word to someone who has had a bad day can make all the difference in the world. My dear sweet mother told me all the time that you can kill more flies with honey. Meditation can make you feel so much more positive and give you a different outlook on life in general, it is something very positive you can do to help yourself.

What she meant was if you have been around someone that wasn't pleasant or had a bad attitude don't act like that person does, instead just turn the other cheek and it may rub off on the person who has a bad attitude. Meditation could be the key to this happening. So you see meditation can be used to turn bad situations into something good or even good situations into something great. Shining the light of the new understanding on those events that happened in the past will help you have a feeling of acceptance, peace,and happiness.

OVERCOMING OBSTACLES WITH MEDITATION

One of the greatest obstacles between you and your happiness is simply one word,stress. By stress I mean a feeling that you have in your mind of fear,anxiety,distress, worry,unease,or foreboding caused by using your mind to imagine a bad outcome to a past,present,or future event.You can use meditation to control your thoughts and feelings. You have to remember things are just things,events are merely events,situations either good or bad are just situations. Its up to you to choose how you will react to the situation, meditation can help you.

Stress will never be completely gone in our lives because of all the negative feedback we have taken on,but by meditating we can eliminate the majority of it.The hard part to eliminate stress is controlling our imaginations to have a happy outcome rather than a poor one.You create your world by your own expectations,and you can influence your future by how you react to the present.If,as part of your meditation,you believe that every event will turn out to be to your benefit,stress will never enter into the picture.

I have spent a lot of time convincing people how meditation can change their lives.When they finally come to believe it,stress was was largely gone from their lives.Many of those whose lives had been nearly ruined by a numerous amount of stress said that using meditation was the greatest gift that they have received.I know meditation is not a gift,but knowing how to control the stress in my life was just like the greatest gift I ever had.If you always remember to stay control of your thoughts,it will be near impossible to feel fear or stress.

You should get a great deal of comfort from the meditation because your imagination is entirely under your control.You have every situation in your life under your control.You can choose to control a bad situation or to turn the bad situation into a better situation. If you are still allowing the events that happened to you to still bother you meditation will not help you.You have to open your mind to understand how meditating will help you.You have got to get all the bad thoughts and anger you feel out of your mind before you start to use meditation.

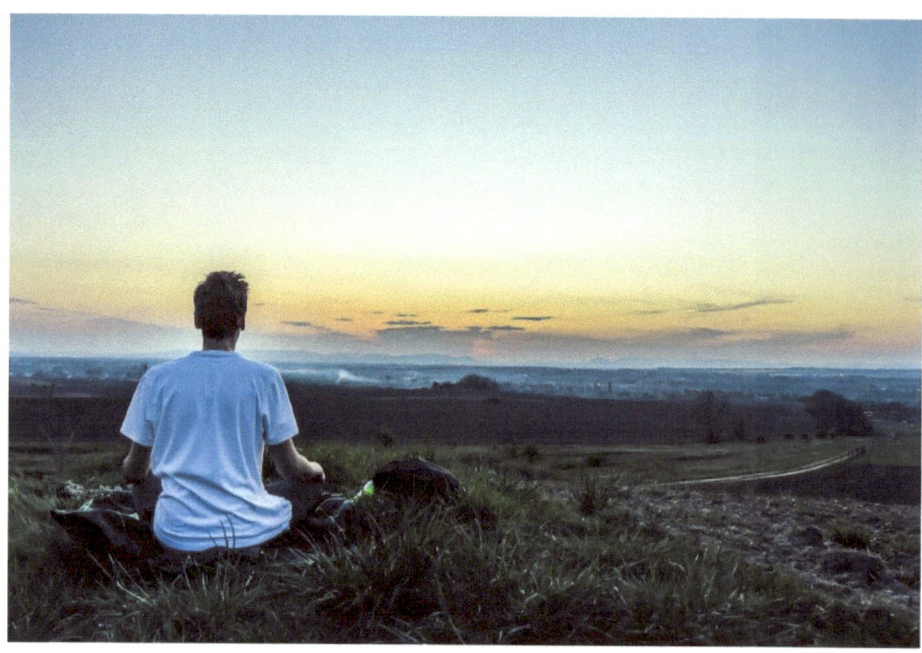

Do something that you feel good about or something that could make you so relaxed that you will let nothing bother you.Once you can allow yourself to relax and feel good about yourself you will see that you than can meditate about the good things that occurred in your day instead of thinking about the things that happened during the day that upset you that you cannot change.

Meditation can help to clear your mind and give you such a relaxing feeling inside, which so many more people should try and conquer throughout their lives. This is something that is not harmful to you in any way and all you have to look forward to from here is living a much less stressful life and feeling better each day when you first step out of bed.

FINDING RELIEF WITH MEDITATION

I would like to take you beyond the limits of your customary thoughts and experiences.This new way of life begins with two questions that are very simple.The first question is would I want this to be true: "Every event that will befall me is absolutely the best possible event that could occur." Meditate before answering this so that you can think about it with a clear mind and answer it truthfully. The second question is the more difficult part,is to truthfully answer this question: Will I give that a chance to be true?

Imagine using meditation that God has appeared before you this instant and said: "I promise you that everything that happens to you from this moment forward will be of the greatest benefit to you and will bring you the utmost good fortune," Suppose God went on to tell you,"Even though what happens will appear at times unfortunate or even hurtful,in the end your life will be wonderfully blessed and hugely benefited by whatever may happen to you.Stop and meditate.How would you feel about that wonderful news? Happy? Perhaps you may even be filled with joy.

Wouldn't it be the greatest news that you could ever hear? Wouldn't you heave a deep sigh of relief and feel as if a great burden had been lifted from your shoulders? Wouldn't you then respond to the next thing that happened-even if it was hurtful or took something from you or seemed bad or even unlucky-as though it was going to be wonderfully beneficial for you,the best possible thing that could have happened? If you have not enthusiastically answer yes,clear your mind,meditate on it.Perhaps you mistaken what I am talking to you about.

I am not talking to you about the common phrase we commonly hear, "try to make the best of things," which basically means " The situation or event really is bad and terribly unlucky, but do what you can possibly think of or meditate to salvage some good out of it." Nor do I mean that within even the worst event possible, there can be found a tiny bit of good. I am not thinking in terms of such limited ideas. I am thinking in unlimited terms, where every event that befalls you is absolutely the best event that could occur-that there is no other event imaginable that could benefit you to any greater degree.

So, again, while you meditate ask yourself wouldn't that be the best piece of news you could hear? If you are willing to give this new concept a chance and actually believe that everything that happens to you will happen for a reason. When thinking about anything, to get a great deal of relief just clear your mind and meditate about the good things that are to come to you in the future. Meditation can be much better than medication and you might just be real surprised how much better you will begin feeling after practicing it for awhile.

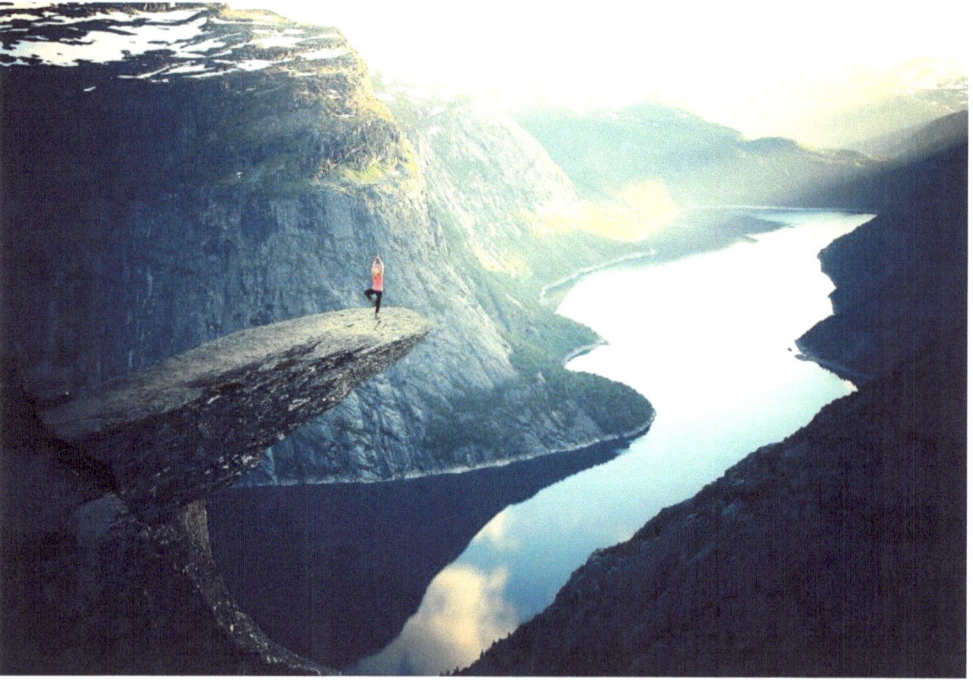

USING MEDITATION THROUGH MUSIC

Clearing your mind through meditation is one of the most peaceful ways you can find to just relieve all the tension you have in your body. Once your mind and body are relaxed you can start to just enjoy some time to yourself. I know that most of us listen to the radio at some point of the day. You may enjoy music ranging from country,to easy listening,to disco,soft rock,classic country,or even blue grass.

Whatever kind of music you enjoy you can find this as a very relaxing way of meditation. For a lot of you that are in good physical shape and like to exercise in a gym at home or even by jogging you want to be able to free your mind of a lot of things that have bothered you through the day.If you are out and about doing your exercises take a Walkman with you and just put it on a station that you really like and let the music just relax all of your tension.

If you are at home exercising or even cooking or cleaning if you have a CD player get one of your favorite Cd's and play it while you are doing the things you need to do.You can also just go get some blank tapes and record your favorite music off the radio for your meditation. One of the things I find relaxing is listening to music while I am working on the computer.

I have found free sites such as lime wire and frost wire and have taken the time to download my all time favorite songs. I transfer the songs I enjoy into my windows media player and play my music everyday when I am on the computer. I just quietly sing along to my favorite music relax and just meditate about my day. I actually use my keyboard a lot and have to do a lot of typing about different subjects. I have found that if I am not completely relaxed and my mind clear I will make many mistakes in my work which I can't afford to do.

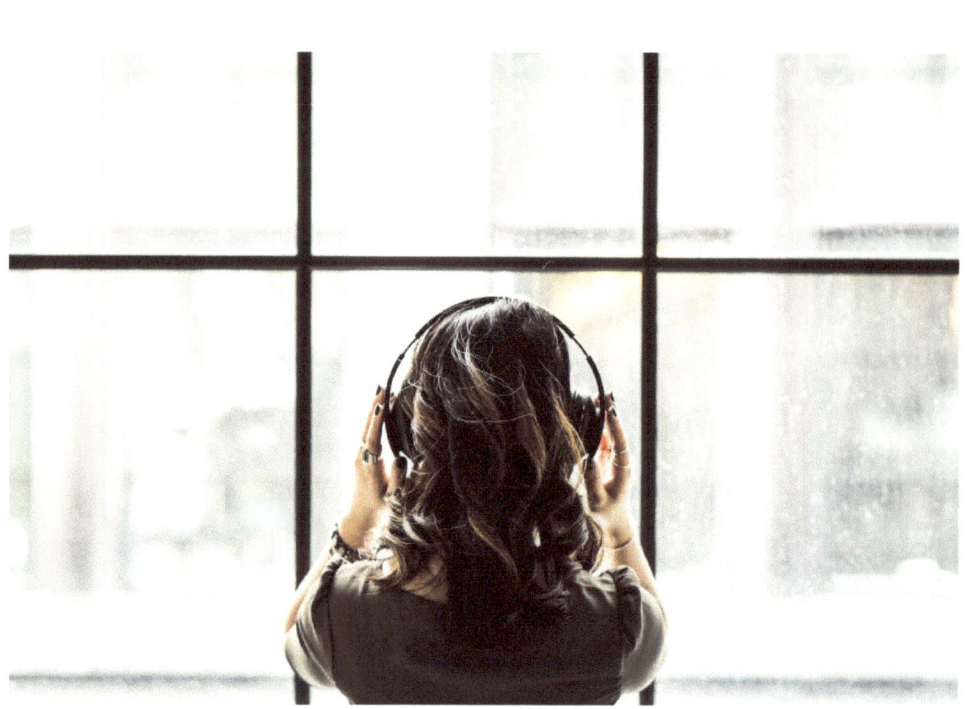

I know I need to be completely relaxed so I pull up my windows media player and play my most favorite songs that will help me to use mediation to get my work done. I have also bought some blank Cd's and burned my favorite songs and then listen to that CD while working on the computer or even going somewhere in my car. After having a busy long hard day and I know I still have to drive home and start my routine of cooking,helping kids with homework,giving the kids a bath and getting them to bed.

As soon as I get in my car and I think about all the things I will have to do I put my CD in the player clear my mind and relax and meditate. After I get all my work done I put the kids to bed and the house is very quiet I will draw me a hot bubble bath and listen to my music and just clear my mind and gather my thoughts so I then can start the next day with a clear head.

So whether you enjoy meditating by exercising,shopping,or listening to your favorite music you will find once you have released all of your tension you can then start to feel good about yourself and when you feel good about yourself you can then feel good about your life.

STOP SMOKING THROUGH MEDITATION

Both self-help groups and clinics offer the quit smoking support programs. Most of these programs are run by professionals and can be customized to meet your needs. You can either attend an intensive quit smoking support program that runs for a week to fifteen days or enroll yourself for weekly sessions.

The popularity of the quit smoking support programs is mainly due to the extensive counseling that they provide to smokers. They teach you to deal with withdrawal symptoms. Meditation can help.

They also provide you support and guidance at every step by understanding your problems. You can talk with the counselors even after you have finished the program. This can help prevent a relapse.

Besides counseling, most quit smoking support programs also prescribe nicotine replacement therapy or NRT. Some also suggest medication like Zyban. Meditation is that experience where one's consciousness becomes engrossed and merged with the object of meditation.

You can also choose from alternative treatments like hypnosis procedures, acupressure and meditation though these are often not very successful. Do what works best to help you to stop smoking, that is what is so very important.

Zyban creates a false feeling of pleasure in the person, a feeling that is similar to the one experienced while smoking. This drug should be taken strictly under medical supervision. It has a few side effects associated with it, and should be avoided by people suffering from heart disease, epilepsy and pregnant women.Beginning with the toes on your left foot, tense the muscles in those toes for a count of three, then slowly release the tension in the toes, and feel a calm return to the toe area. You need support during this difficult time so please talk with someone about it who can provide you with that help.

Do the same with the toes on the right foot.

Since the chances of a relapse are very high, most quit smoking support programs have a 24-hour help line service where counselors listen to queries and provide solutions. At the end of a program the smokers are given listening and reading material to reinforce their resolve to quit smoking.

Quit smoking support can also be extended by friends and family members. They can play a big role in keeping their friend or relative occupied. They can also help in preventing relapse by urging the smokers to return to the quit smoking support program if the need arises.

The advantage with NRT is that it reduces your craving for nicotine. You can use NRT in the form of gums, patches, sprays and inhalers. Though gums and patches are available over the counter other forms of NRT can be taken only under medical supervision. They reduce your nicotine dependency by releasing a small quantity of nicotine into the body. The dosage can be regulated to control the withdrawal symptoms, and stopped completely once your urge to smoke disappears.

Meditation can help.Good luck on your way to a new fresh non smoking world, you are really going to love it.

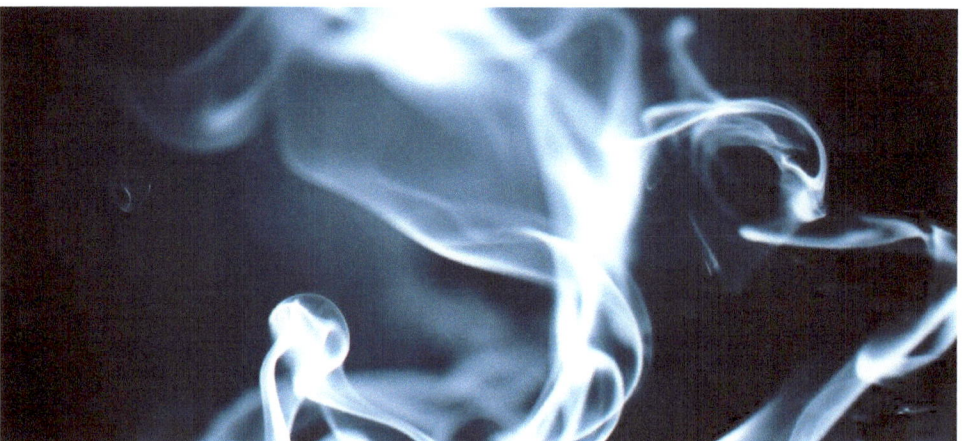

CREATING NEW EXPERIENCES THROUGH MEDITATION

How can you change what you believe when the experiences you have had has convinced you otherwise? The simple answer to that is to create a new experience. The best way for you to get that new experience is to meditate about how you can change the way you respond to what happens. The new response will create new results, which you will then experience it as a new reality.

To reach your goal of happiness, you have to act as though the following statement is true: Everything that happens to me is the best possible thing that can happen to me. meditating to help turn a bad situation into something good can be as easy as: 1+ 1 = 2. Acting as though what happens to you is the best possible thing that can happen to you plus the new results just equals happiness in your life.

When you are convinced of the truth that everything that happens is the best thing that can happen, life will Begin to be much more fun. It is like opening a new channel to happiness. All you need to know when meditating is happiness is there, waiting just for you. All you need to do is follow the formula that creates it. You have to remember also that unhappiness is also out there, waiting just for you.

The way you respond through meditation will determine which one you will be experiencing in your life. It is not necessary to have all the ingredients of a project in hand at the outset. They will come at the appointed time. It's only important that you move forward with the project that you have started until that appointed time comes. With the energy you create through meditation by moving forward as if you had the money to start your project, you actually put into motion a start of events that will lead you to your success.

Your actions create an energy that draws in the necessary ingredients of your project you have ventured into. Everything that you need for your venture is, in actuality, already out there, waiting for you. You only need to draw in what is needed. There is really nothing more to all of this other than just you remembering to keep an open mind and find that peace that is buried deep within you.

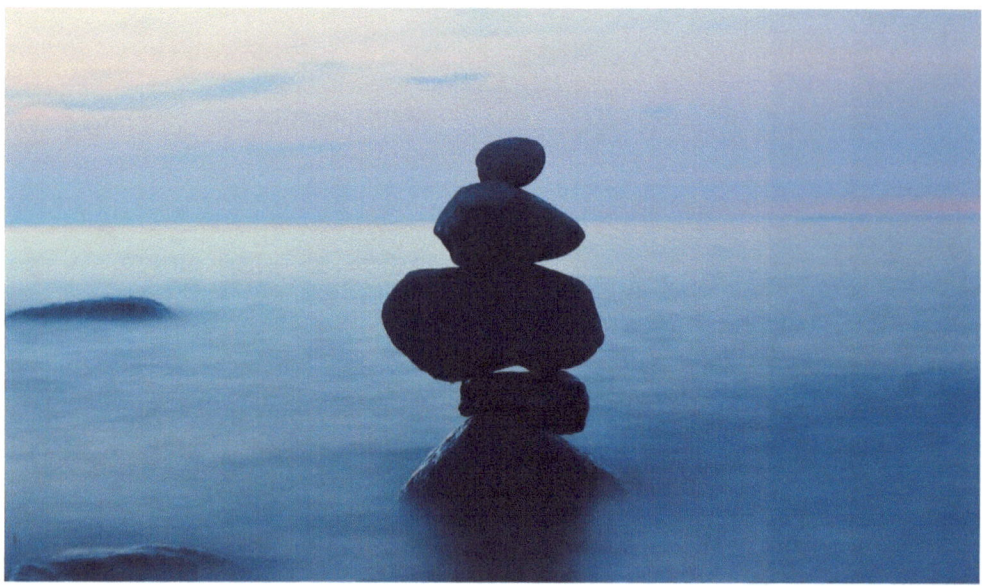

The result that come with meditation that causes you to experience happiness,which then proves to you that this is how things really do work-and this leads you to soon believe that everything does indeed happen for your benefit. When you realize that is true,that is when the deep sighs of relief will come and that meditation can certainly help you see the light.

The internet is a really great place to find out all of the information that you would need about meditation, in case you are interested in learning more about it for your own benefits. This is very important for you to consider doing because it will relieve you from so much stress circulating throughout your life each and everyday. Try practicing meditation as often as you can because you are really going to benefit from it.

ADAPTING TO CHANGE BY MEDITATION

Adapting to any kind of change in your life can be very stressful. The one thing I have learned when it comes to any kind of change is to keep it on a positive level. To do that I stay calm by meditating and keep it all in perspective. I was talking to a friend how I was very apprehensive about a change I would soon have to make in my life.She told me that almost over twenty years ago she had bought a brand new car and it was parked in an alley next to her house.

She walked out of the house just in time to see and old vw bus scrape the front fender of her car. As she continued to tell me what happened she let me know she was trying to stay calm and knew she had to meditate and get focused on the situation. She went on to tell me that the driver got out of his car,threw his hat on the ground,then hung his head,holding it in his hands. She knew that he obviously didn't have the money to pay for the damage to her car and he almost started to cry.

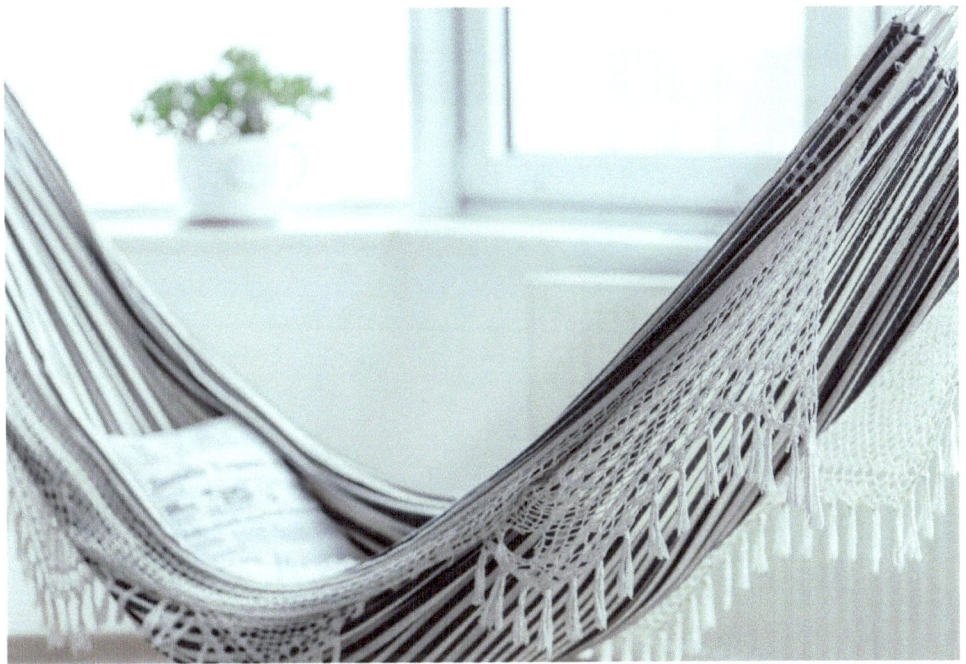

My friend still meditating to keep things in perspective walked up to the man and you could tell he was very nervous and expected her to say something like What an idiot, Are you blind, or just something so mean that he would just feel terrible. As she walked up to the man she simply said don't worry about the scrape and to have a nice day. He couldn't believe what he was hearing. He began to cry tears of happiness and hugged my friend. He then ran to his wife who was in the car wondering what they were going to do and he hugged his wife and introduced her to my friend.

As they were talking my friend told them how she used meditation to keep as calm as possible because she had a temper in the past that caused her a lot of problems. The man and his wife and my friend became the best of friends. Here it is 20 years later and even though the man has now passed away and his wife is in a home for the elderly my friend still visits the woman every week and still talk about the day they had met.

Using meditation will certainly help you think about the situation your in and to not act on impulse, but to handle whatever situation it is you are in you will act responsibly. After my friend and I talked I thought how I could adapt to the change I would have to make by positive thinking and could make a bad situation into something that will have a very special meaning in my life. After our talk I went home and started using meditation to relax myself and now I feel better about

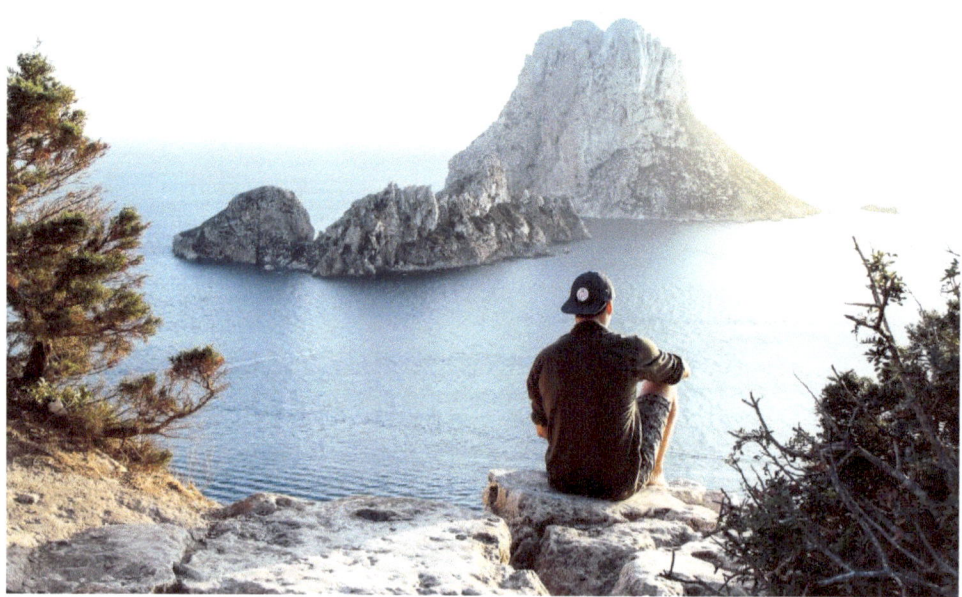

CONTROLLING ANGER BY MEDITATION

I have never really thought of myself as an angry person.I would always do whatever I could to try and help someone out,nor did I do anything that would hurt someones feelings,or I would try as hard as I could not to. Every month we struggle to get by but I really didn't complain. I was just happy that we did have the money to pay our bills and have a place to live even though we barely had enough to survive on after paying the bills. Meditation is very much needed in most peoples lives, no doubt about that.

Even after all that I did not get angry,That changed last week.I really had to meditate to myself when I went with my sister to the doctor last week.My sister is a very hard worker.She never misses work unless it is absolutely necessary.Last year my sister had become sick and finally after being so weak she went to the doctor.He put her in the hospital and gave her 4 bags of blood and said she had pneumonia.

I just couldn't understand how do you lose blood by having pneumonia.As I meditated thinking about last year I was not prepared to hear what the doctor was going to say as my sister and I were driving to the doctor.You see my sister got sick again. She nearly collapsed at work and was taken to the hospital.This time she needed 5 bags of blood.She would keep telling me she was anemic.After the hospital did a ct scan on her they said she needed to go to her lung doctor immediately.That's where my sister and I were going.

My sister never wants me to worry so she never told me anything and did not want me to go in the room with her when she went in to see the doctor.After I meditated on this I decided when they called her name I would go back with her,and that's exactly what I did.The doctor came in and you could see immediately the concern on his face.He starting reading the results of her ct scan.He was reading something about her lungs.

He talked about something growing in her nodules and spreading to her lymph nodes.He wasn't saying it was cancer but I knew by what he was reading it was. I didn't want to scare my sister so meditating to myself while he was talking I asked what does all this mean? Instead of asking is it cancer I asked could it be cancer?

His response was yes mam.She has to go for a biopsy in a couple of days to see how far it has progressed.I really find myself angry at this point because she has never smoked a day in her life,And here she is 49 years old with lung cancer.So instead of worrying for the next couple of days and getting angry,I simply practice meditation by praying that god please heal my sister.

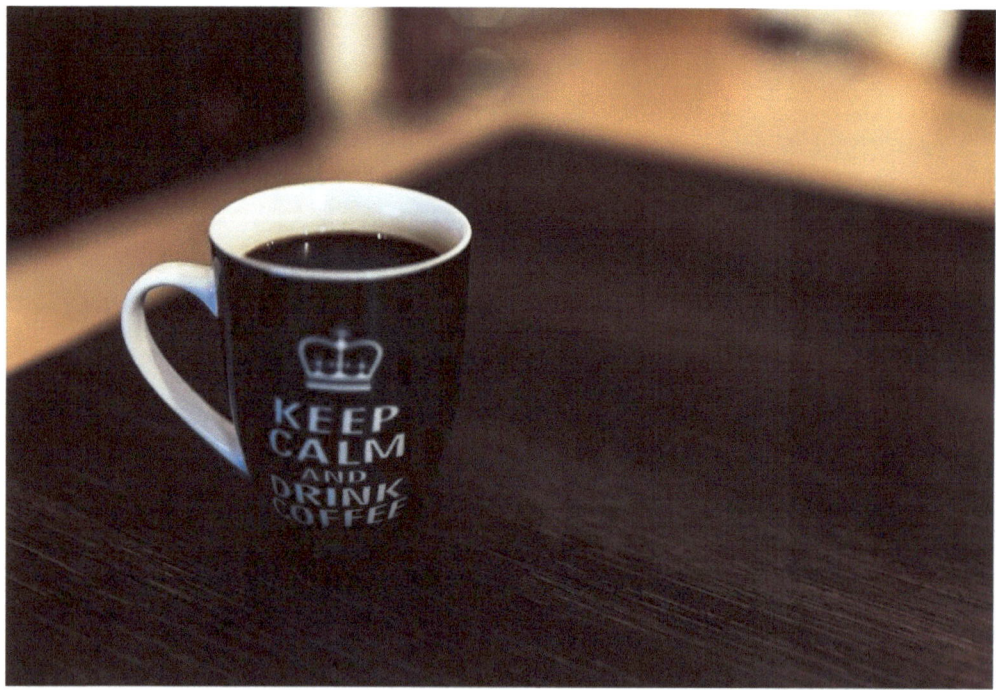

DIFFERENT AND HELPFUL THINGS TO KNOW ABOUT MEDITATION

Relaxation techniques are a great way to help your pursuit to reduce stress. Relaxation isn't just about peace of mind or enjoying a hobby. Relaxation is a process that decreases the wear and tear of life's challenges on your mind and body. Whether you have a lot of stress in your life or you've got it under control, you can benefit from learning relaxation techniques. Learning basic meditation relaxation techniques isn't hard.

Explore these simple relaxation techniques to get you started on de-stressing your life and improving your health.
There are ample of sources of stress in the world now a days. As the old saying goes, "there's no need to look for trouble, because trouble will find you all on its own". All of us have troubles and worries, along with all these stresses, few of us even have time to kick back and relax. If you suffer from anxiety and did you wish to ease that anxious moods you have and feel relax for a while?

There are number of relaxations techniques you have that you take a little time and are highly effective which you can done anywhere even at work.
If I were to find a perfect relaxation techniques I would preferred to make a fortune sharing with others. In this, there are a lot of great ideas, and these ideas published in different places but it seems no one got it gold. I know that the people around me seem to be more and more stressed as time goes along. More people tried many relaxation techniques but they only find nothing work for them.

There are many different things you can try, but you may have to search for a while before you find something that works for you.
Performing breathing can be therapeutic, and with enough practice, can become your standard way of breathing. To breathe with the diaphragm, one must draw air into the lungs in a way which will expand the stomach and not the chest.

It is best to perform these breaths as long, slow intakes of air - allowing the body to absorb all of the inhaled oxygen while simultaneously relaxing the breather. To do this comfortably, it is often best to loosen tight-fitting pants, belts, skirts as these can interfere with the body's ability to intake air. The old-fashioned remedy of breathing slowly into a paper bag works amazingly well to relax you and restore proper breathing. Another version of this relaxation technique involves taking slow deep breaths. At first you may find you need to force yourself to breathe slowly, but persist and you'll soon be back to normal.

And bear in mind that some people, especially those with significant psychological problems and a history of abuse, may experience feelings of emotional discomfort during relaxation exercises. Although this is rare, if you experience emotional discomfort during relaxation exercises, stop what you're doing and consider talking to your health care professional. Some relaxation techniques will work for some people, while some will leave others feeling cold. Write down all of your ideas and move through your list one at a time. This may help you find relaxation techniques that work best for you and your lifestyle.

I know that the people around me seem to be more and more stressed as time goes along. More people tried many relaxation techniques but they only find nothing work for them. There are many different things you can try, but you may have to search for a while before you find something that works for you.
Performing breathing can be therapeutic, and with enough practice, can become your standard way of breathing.

To breathe with the diaphragm, one must draw air into the lungs in a way which will expand the stomach and not the chest. It is best to perform these breaths as long, slow intakes of air - allowing the body to absorb all of the inhaled oxygen while simultaneously relaxing the breather. To do this comfortably, it is often best to loosen tight-fitting pants, belts, skirts as these can interfere with the body's ability to intake air.

The old-fashioned remedy of breathing slowly into a paper bag works amazingly well to relax you and restore proper breathing. Another version of this relaxation technique involves taking slow deep breaths. At first you may find you need to force yourself to breathe slowly, but persist and you'll soon be back to normal. Meditation can help you throughout your entire life.

DIFFERENT FORMS OF MEDITATION

There are no special tricks to meditating; no special posture or breathing rhythm is required. Once you have gotten the knack of it you can meditate anywhere during any activity. Some readers have succeeded in reaching this altered state of conscious while reading about my sand meditation, perhaps you too may realize this transformational state of consciousness as you read on…

Sometimes meditation opens a door into the mysteries of creation. If we allow ourselves to pass through this door there is no telling what we may encounter on the other side. Do not become discouraged if you have tried to meditate in the past and not gotten any remarkable results. Meditation is a mystical process and it may take awhile to learn how to quiet your mind and open yourself to all the present moment has to offer you.

My meditation began while sitting on a beach. My hands were sandy. I rubbed my thumb and forefinger together feeling the grains of sand between them slipping away until only a single grain of sand remained.
I could feel the shape of the grain of sand distinctly as I rolled it back and forth between my thumb and forefinger.

The longer I rolled the grain of sand about the more defined my awareness of the grain of sand became. The more detailed my experience of the grain of sand became the larger it appeared to be.
While I could clearly feel the tiny grain of sand trapped between my thumb and finger roll about across the grooves and ridges of my fingerprints the grain of sand appeared to be growing larger and larger as I contemplated it.

The grain of sand continued to grow, encompassing the beach and then the world. Before long the grain of sand had grown to an infinite size and it now encompassed all of creation; yet I still held the tiny grain of sand between my thumb and forefinger, rolling it about across the grooves and ridges of my fingerprints.

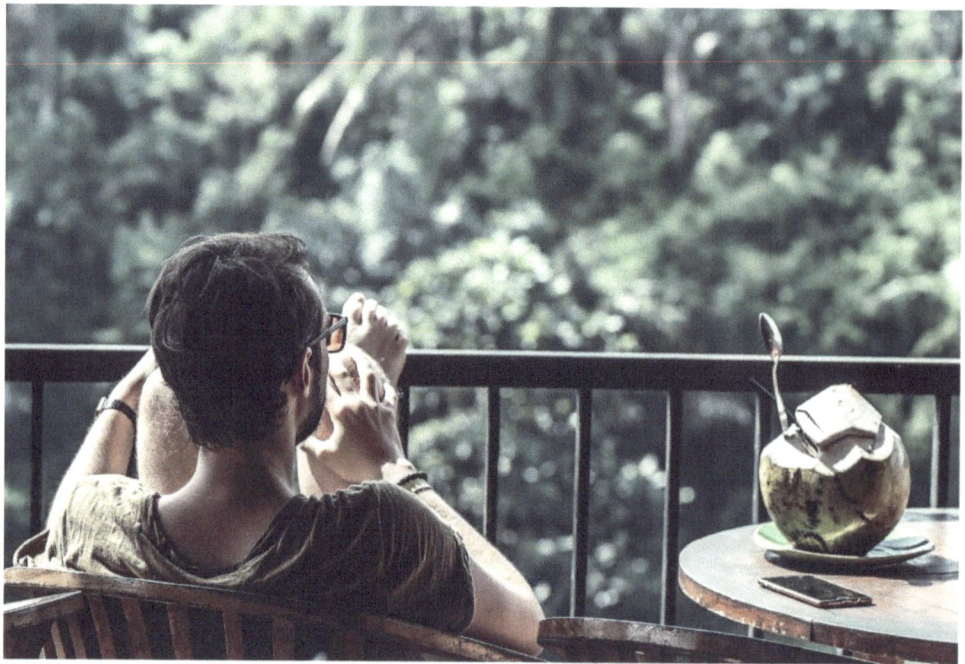

The tiny grain of sand was intimately connected to every part of creation and all of creation existed within it, even as it existed within my grasp. I communed with the grain of sand, aware of its infinite connectedness to everything else; through the medium of the grain of sand I became aware of my own infinite connectedness with all of creation.

The sand spoke to me of eternity. It told me tales about creation and the infinite nature of our existence in creation. From the grain of sand I learned that every tiniest part of creation is a living being experiencing creation and sharing in the process whereby creation makes everything manifest.

My meditation with a grain of sand always produced a feeling of intense bliss. It was an eternal meditation that transcended the time and place where it began to continue throughout all of creation. From time to time I would return to this meditation, engrossed by the wisdom and experience of a single tiny grain of sand.

ACHIEVING HAPPINESS THROUGH MEDITATION

There is only one way to achieve happiness. That way is to simply be happy. You are probably thinking right now how do i get to be happy." "Things just don't work like that, It doesn't take into consideration the times that I am miserable because of problems or mishaps that come up in my everyday life, not to mention the tragedies." At this point I have to stop and meditate. Meditation can be done many different ways, just find the one that works best for your purposes.

Being happy much more of the time than you have been is an incredibly difficult task to accomplish-not in the doing of it once you know how and then in keeping aware of what you have discovered. Yet, I still say that with meditation you can do it. The path that you have chose that led you to your current situation was not a few days or months in the making, but a long and strenuous path that has spanned through many years.

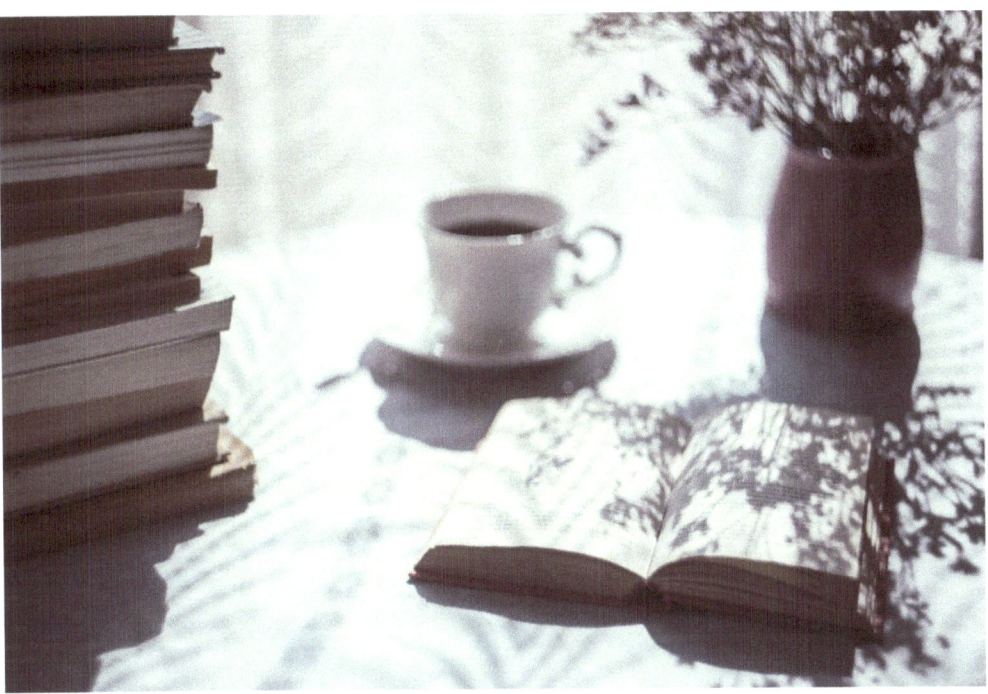

There is only one way to achieve happiness.That way is to simply be happy.You are probably thinking right now how do i get to be happy." "Things just don't work like that, It doesn't take into consideration the times that I am miserable because of problems or mishaps that come up in my everyday life,not to mention the tragedies." At this point I have to stop and meditate. Meditation can be done many different ways, just find the one that works best for your purposes.

Being happy much more of the time than you have been is an incredibly difficult task to accomplish-not in the doing of it once you know how and then in keeping aware of what you have discovered.Yet,I still say that with meditation you can do it.The path that you have chose that led you to your current situation was not a few days or months in the making,but a long and strenuous path that has spanned through many years.

In reality it has taken you as long as you have been alive to become the way you are today.It has also taken you that long to achieve what you have achieved, to possess,and to arrive at your current condition.By taking the time to meditate and think about who you are,and what you have in your life is truly what you want,If you are completely satisfied with the way your life is going,congratulations-do more of what you have been doing and you will get more of what you already have in your life.

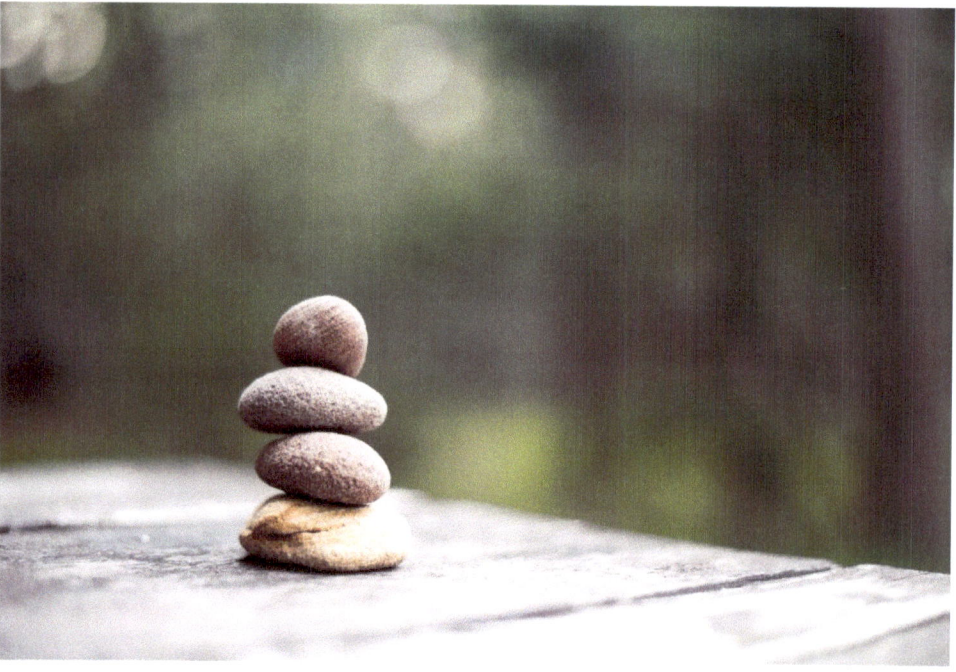